Golfer's Elbow & Tennis Elbow explained.

Golfer's Elbow / Tennis Elbow /
Epicondylitis Treatment, Exercises,
Symptoms, Causes, Surgery, Cure, Braces,
Relief and Remedies all covered.

by

Robert Rymore

Published by IMB Publishing 2013

Table of Contents

Table Of Contents

Disclaimer

This disclaimer serves to announce that this book was written by the author as a reader's guide to provide education on epicondylitis. We believe the information contained herein to be accurate and current, though neither the author nor the publisher accept any legal accountability for the authenticity, quality and welfare of information found in this book.

Website, service provider, product or manufacturer mentioned in this book serve the purpose of knowledge exchange and do not establish approval, confirmation, favor and or certification by the author and or publisher.

Epicondylitis is a reader's guide and is not an alternative to medical consultation, diagnosis and treatment. Any consequences resulting due to a breach in the terms of its use herein enclosed is not a responsibility of the author and any affiliated entities. Using this guide as a medical consulting platform is prohibited.

Additionally, distribution of any copyrighted material from this book without agreement or consent from the copyright owner is strictly illegal.

Acknowledgments

I am indebted to Jasmine Fowler for her valuable suggestions and support in completing this endeavor. Appreciation goes to Lorna Preston for decrypting my somewhat difficult handwriting to a superb typed version. It is also my privilege to express gratitude to Esther Hewlett, Fatima Armin and Jeremy Clark for wonderful suggestions and exceptional editing. Also, recognition goes to my family, for their never-ending support and encouragement without which this would not have been possible. To my long-term publisher who for many years has professionally delivered, thank you.

Thanks to my wife and children for supporting me.

Chapter 1) What is epicondylitis?

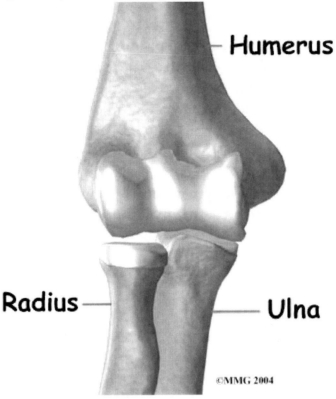

Humerus

Radius

Ulna

©MMG 2004

If you bend your elbow halfway through and palpate on its sides, the bony prominences you feel are epicondyles. Epicondyles are bony protrusions that serve a purpose of muscle tendon attachment. The bony protuberance on the side of the elbow which touches the chest when you squeeze the armpit tight is the inner (medial) humeral epicondyle while the one further is the outer (lateral) humeral epicondyle. Humerus is the long bone in between the shoulder and the elbow, where at the elbow it widens like a knob to form the elbow joint as it articulates with 2 other bones, the radius and the ulna.

During growth and maturation of the skeletal system, bone remodeling is governed by Wolff's Law, a theory which a German anatomist and surgeon developed in the 19th century. It states that if loading on a particular bone increases, the bone remodels over time to become stronger, hence to better suit the sort of loading exerted upon it. With daily strenuous activities, great force is exerted on the elbow, thus more bone is laid down on that zone to resist the high force applied, forming epicondyles.

The forearm, the region between the elbow and the wrist, consists of 2 muscle groups. Those that extend the wrist and the fingers (extensors), like in an upward movement to throttle a motorcycle, while flexors flex the wrist and fingers like in dunking a basket at a basketball game. Muscles of the forearm have an origin, the point where they are initially attached, and an insertion, the site where their end attachment is located. All the extensors of the wrist have one origin point, where tendons of these extensors attach to the bony prominence of the lateral epicondyle. Tendons are thick fibrous bands, which connect a locomotive muscle to a bone, acting as a pulley system to transmit forces from muscles into the bone bringing about movement by the displacement of the bone in the required direction. Overuse by repetitive activities, like overhead arm movements, can cause micro trauma and inflammation of these tendons, a process which is called tendonitis, interchangeably used with tendinitis, though having the same meaning. There is a need to differentiate tendonitis from tendinosis, which is degenerative deterioration of a tendon. Degeneration consisting of cellular component reduction, vascular compromise, reduction in elasticity and tendon strength leaving tendons vulnerable to repetitive stress injuries (RSIs). Epicondylitis is thus a type of tendonitis, though not exclusively as it has a combined effect with that of tendinosis. Lateral epicondylitis is also called tennis elbow because it has been a diagnosis mostly found in tennis players, due to their repetitive upward arm movements during serving and tennis racket swing movements, especially the backhand. 10% of all lateral epicondylitis have actually been shown to have occurred in tennis-associated tendon injuries. On the contrary, medial epicondylitis, also termed golfer's elbow, is not a strict golf player's condition. Flexors of the forearm originate on the medial epicondyle. Repeated excessive stress which is constantly being exerted on the flexor tendons results in medial epicondylitis, (this reference to flexor tendons, is directed in particular to the flexor carpi radialis, a specific muscle belly you palpate or see when your forearm is extended in front, with a formed fist facing up, moving the fist up and down in an effort to touch the forearm). Of all golfer's elbows we have dealt with, none have ever actually been caused by playing golf. Golfer's elbow does occur because of wrist flexion overuse activities associated with sporting and recreational activities, among which are fastball pitching and canoeing, as well as occupational injuries especially in people who have flexor tendon stresses with an addition of vibration, in which concrete drilling and mining is mentioned. Golfers however, often suffer from shoulder tendonitis (rotator cuff).

Tennis elbow is a frequent diagnosis in comparison to golfer's elbow, though in general, epicondylitis is a frequent diagnosis.

Chapter 2) Anatomy

a) The elbow

Careful evaluation of the elbow is important to differentiate epicondylitis from pain and tenderness occurring due to other causes, which can be in any category among bone, ligament, nerves, vessels, muscles and joint injuries, or disease. This portrays a need for understanding the elbow and its associated pathologies, without which a correct diagnosis of epicondylitis can be easily missed.

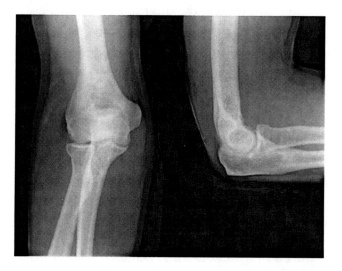

The elbow is a hinge joint made up of the humerus, ulna and radius. Imagining a door hinge, movement of the elbow can be in an upward flexion movement as in moving the hand to touch the ipsilateral shoulder and downward extension movement as in placing the forearm straight with palms facing up. A little rotation is possible at the elbow joint because of the unique positioning and interaction of the bones that form it. The bones of the elbow

11

are stabilized first by its structure, having a partial lock and key where one bone sits into another. Ligaments, fibrous protein bands connecting bone to bone, positioned on the lateral and medial sides of the elbow, are continuous with the joint capsule to form a very strong fibrous capsule covering the elbow joint. The joint capsule, together with ligaments, prevent over-gliding of the articulating bones in any direction, which can result in a partial disposition of the bones, what is termed sublaxation of a joint or a total displacement known as a dislocation. Inside the joint capsule is a fluid-producing membrane, synovium, which produces a lubricating synovial fluid for friction-free mobility. Muscles covering the elbow joint also protect the joint by cushion. These are elbow flexors, in particular the bicep muscle, wrist flexors, flexor carpi radialis, extensors of the elbow and wrist extensors such as extensor carpi radialis brevis (ECRB). Bursae, small synovial fluid-producing sacs found under tendons, allow smooth movement of the tendon against the bone, protecting it from friction rub that can result in wearing off of a tendon leading to failure of the system. Blood vessels and nerves also pass by the joint, providing adequate blood supply with nutrients and oxygen for cell metabolism and growth, with innervation and sensation completing the true picture of a normal healthy elbow.

Changes in any of the elbow joint-stabilizing substances result in pathology of the joint, athropathy, athro- meaning joint and - pathy for pathology. Athropathy, regardless of the cause, results in loss of function, especially if it occurs on the main limb, of right-handedness or left-handedness. Epicondylitis among other athropathies require one to be competent in general elbow examination and in particular trick tests and tips to confirm the diagnosis.

Athritis, inflammation of a joint, of the synovium, synovitis are main complaints of the elbow usually in the elderly with degenerative joint diseases and chondropathies. Infection, fracture, dislocation, tendonitis and bursitis being the other cadres. Peripheral neuropathies are uncommon, with ulnar nerve compression syndrome (cubital syndrome), being at the top of the list because of the ulnar nerve position at the elbow joint, which is situated in a groove behind the medial epicondyle, the ulnar groove. Pain at the elbow is a puzzle, which requires experience and proper knowledge if a correct treatment plan is to be initiated.

Pathology at the elbow can be acute or chronic. Acute is defined as a pathology lasting a short period of time of 3weeks or less, beyond which it becomes chronic. Epicondylitis is usually of the chronic type, partly because of inadequate treatment plans that offer temporary relief and poor sporting techniques that even in an attempt to heal micro trauma by the tendon, more torture is entrusted upon it again and again. It is thus inevitable that many people with epicondylitis will continue to suffer until a better understanding of the condition, together with its associations, is completely understood by both the sufferer and his or her physician. We currently understand that epicondylitis is the pain and discomfort experienced as a result of an inflamed wrist flexor tendon and/or extensor muscle tendon at its point of origin, the medial or lateral epicondyle, in which inflammation is not a primary culprit, but a combination of events greatly played by tendinosis.

This per se does not mean acute epicondylitis is nonexistent. Usually, it may not be reported as acute epicondylitis, but falls under a different diagnosis. For instance, acute rupture of a tendon, whether partial or total, always causes inflammation of the tendon because it is one of the phases in wound or tissue healing.

Inflammation is therefore indeed a sheep with a fox spirit. In a normal reaction to injury like tendon tear, inflammation occurs to assist the injured site to recruit appropriate cells, energy, nutrients, blood supply and blood clotting factors together with immunological substances all for the sole purpose of initiating wound and/or tissue repair. In another scenario, inflammation in epicondylitis has the same process of recruiting cells and other substances, though in an attempt to heal cause further damage by inadequate healing and improper, rather excessive fibrous tissue build up on tendons. This reduces an otherwise slightly elastic recoiling quality of tendons to a stiff, non stretchable material which fails with time. A partial or total tear is inevitable upon overstretch and overuse, that also being the reason why tendon rupture is the leading complication in tendonitis and of interest epicondylitis.

b) Tendon

Epicondylitis is an overuse injury to tendons of the elbow. The main question is, what makes a tendon? Why are they vulnerable to injuries? Is it their anatomical makeup? What then is their anatomy? Here is an overview of what makes up a tendon.

Within the human body, strength of a tissue depends on its components, blood supply, its function and repair strategies. Likewise, tendons are peculiar in their makeup and blood supply. A tendon is a thick fibrous band made up of collagen fibrils and fibers interwoven together to form a single highly resistant rope. Collagen occupies 30% of the dry mass of a tendon and is a protein found in 30% of the entire human body. Collagen is found in ligaments, tendons, bones, cartilage and skin, giving shape and strength to these structures. Many types of collagen exist; a total of 29 different kinds are known and their use in tissues is dependent upon genetic selection. In tendons, type I collagen is abundant, but other types such as types III and IV are also present in meager quantities. In between collagen fibers, the so called extracellular matrix, are proteoglycans, glycoproteins, an elastic substance called elastin, cells such as tenoblasts and tenocytes. Tenocytes are mature tenoblasts responsible for collagen molecule production. Collagen molecules conglomerate to form fibrils, which join further to form fibers. These fibers intertwine together to form the well–known, three-dimensional collagen structure. A protective sheath called endotenon encircles the 3D fibers. Multiple endotenon-covered fibers form fascicles, which are surrounded by yet another sheath called an epitenon to form the tendon. Some other tendons are covered by a synovial sheath, such as the long head of the biceps tendon. However, this is not the case with flexor and extensor tendons at the elbow. A synovial sheath is a membrane that produces lubricating fluid in the body in areas of high friction, such as joints and the base of tendons. Some specialists consider tendons of the elbow to be a myth, since they lack a gliding mechanism and appear to be musculo-ligamentous intra-operatively or in cadaveric examination.

It is important to know about tendon blood supply, which comes from the bone, muscle and a central tendon supply running in the paratenon. This blood supply is divided into intrinsic and extrinsic - intrinsic being the central supply and extrinsic from bone and muscle. Since tendons are intermediates between muscles and bones, they have to be connected to both. At the tendon-muscular junction, blood vessels from muscles cross over to supply a third of the tendon from that junction. The same applies to the blood supply from the bone-tendon junction, although crossing over of blood vessels to the tendon at this particular junction is limited. This leaves the middle tendon part with the least blood supply, the so-called "watershed zone." It is in this area that most tendon injuries occur. Limited blood supply will mean a slow healing process in case of injury, which is true for tendons. Other weak zones are those where the most tendon-surface friction takes place, an impingement site like that of the supraspinatus muscle in the shoulder or in the case of epicondylitis, where the most stress is exerted.

All this may sound like medical gibberish, but the most important thing is, to know that tendons are made from collagen, cells and other components; that with age tendon components degenerate, cells become fewer, leading to a decrease in extracellular matrix formation; collagen fibers also decrease, their laxity and strength are compromised and generally their healing becomes even worse besides it being usually slow.

The good news is that there is still some hope of relief and a cure when one suffers from tendinopathies such as tennis or golfer's elbow. With the correct treatment programs of inflammation and pain relief, topped off with exercise many have been completely cured for years now. If you are reading this book because you are suffering from epicondylitis, congratulations, you are in luck, for you have come to the right place.

Chapter 3) Are You a Sufferer?

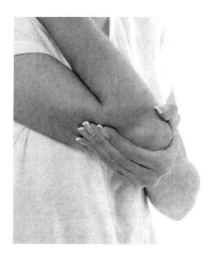

Epicondylitis is common in all individuals, though predominantly in the third to fifth decades of life. In the majority of cases, over 70 percent of epicondylitis occurs in the dominant arm, right or left-handedness. Its distribution is equal among males and females, although distribution changes in specific risk group professions. People whose jobs involve vibration, frequent overhead reaching, awkward positions and forceful exertions are top listing on the epicondylitis diagnosis. Sporting activities that involve repetitive motion, especially if combined with poor technique are included, such as tennis, swimming, golf, bowling, baseball, weightlifting, softball and basketball. Epicondylitis can be caused by a sudden injury, such as a direct bump or hit over the tendon, but almost always occurs over time from the repetition of particular movements and tendinosis. Lifestyle risk factors like smoking, alcohol abuse and a sedentary life have a share of their own in epicondylitis exacerbation. Age contributes a large part to epicondylitis development. Geriatric tendon changes include fewer cells, fibroblasts, which produce connective tissue with an altered component balance forming dense, thickened and contracted tendons, with or without calcification. This scarring forms adhesions, which restrict movement, causing pain and tenderness.

Concomitant disease conditions, where diabetes mellitus, hypertension, arthritis and osteoporosis are the most common, contribute to epicondylitis and tendonitis in general. Aggravations of these disease states and/or their poor control lead to an overall health decline.

Epicondylitis can usually be diagnosed by a careful patient history and physical examination, although a physician may order X-rays and or other imaging tests to differentiate it from other probable elbow diseases.

In the beginning, pain and tenderness may be felt on the outsides of the elbow, with reference down to the wrist along respective muscles - this occurs even at rest. Movement against resistance gives a sharp, excruciating pain and is a diagnostic examination trick. It may occur with daily life activities like lifting a cup of coffee with the elbow pressed on the table.

A little swelling and warmth may be felt on the epicondyles. X-rays are almost always normal, except 20% in which some calcification can be noted at tendon origin sites. MRI can show tears within the tendon and laboratory tests may support other diagnoses like rheumatoid factor for rheumatoid arthritis. Accurate diagnosis of epicondylitis is dependent upon a total understanding of the structure, distribution and pathophysiological factors that distinguish epicondylitis from other elbow conditions, which is why it is necessary to consult your doctor for diagnosis.

Chapter 4) Differential Diagnosis

a) What is DDx?

Differential diagnosis, abbreviated DDx, DD or D/Dx, is distinguishing a disease or condition from other disease states presenting with similar signs and symptoms. This can be made possible by systematically eliminating candidate conditions by taking a careful patient history, epidemiology, performing a complete clinical examination, imaging techniques such as X-rays, MRIs, CT-scans, function evaluation tests such as electromyography, nerve conduction tests and laboratory investigations of blood work which include general full blood picture, biochemistry of electrolytes, and even probability calculations, especially in genetic diseases. Differential diagnosis procedures are used by physicians or trained medical professionals to diagnose the specific disease in a patient or eliminate life-threatening conditions. The first step in differentiating a diagnosis, is knowing possible conditions that exist to a particular set of symptoms. Epicondylitis as an elbow complaint presents with symptoms and signs of many other medical conditions, which can be grouped or classified in many ways. Mnemonics are often used by medical students and physicians to ensure that all possible pathological processes are considered, as they provide an easy, systematic way to remember. For instance, VITAMIN D, which can be expanded to mean: V-vascular, I-Inflammatory, T- Traumatic, A- Autoimmune, M-Metabolic, I- Infectious, N- Neoplasm/Nerves and D-Degenerative. Many other ways exist of tackling differential diagnosis.

In this text, we are going to use differential diagnosis of epicondylitis by stability of the elbow joint as explained in the previous chapter, i.e. bones, joint, ligaments, bursae, muscles, nerves and blood vessels with top listed medical conditions briefly explained for a better understanding.

b) Bones

The elbow, as we understand it, is formed by the humerus, radius and ulna articulating together. These bones can be suffering from an intrinsic disease condition, which can result in pain, tenderness and reduced use of the joint called pseudo paralysis. Bone disease is known as osteopathy and can occur at the elbow if symptoms are to be mistaken for epicondylitis and/or vice versa. It is of importance to note that pain at the elbow does not always originate at the elbow. Referred pain is pain that is felt at another site other than its main source, such as pain in the shoulder being felt at the elbow due to transference along peripheral nerve distribution. These points from which pain can be transferred from are called trigger points and are often at the shoulder. Pain is referred to the elbow from a trigger point, these points have to be located and pressed. If a point is a trigger point, then more pain will be felt at the elbow. Another source of pain can be rotator cuff injury, which is another common tendon injury and is located at the shoulder. Moving the shoulder through full range of motion and doing specific examinations can confirm its presence. Not to mention referred pain from the cervical spine, what is termed radicular pain or radiculopathy. Radiculopathy occurs when the nerves are compressed on their outlets causing pain along the segment supplied by that particular nerve. Compression at the spine can occur from bony spurs, reduced vertebral space and/or disc prolapse. Differentiating radicular pain requires a neck examination by a physician, palpation to check for tender spots on the vertebra and X-rays to show any pathology. A spring test can be done, in standing position with shoulders straight and arms on the sides, turn the head towards the side with affected elbow, stretching the neck slightly further. This will act as compression stimulation and if the pain worsens or appears the test is positive. All these considerations are required to locate the source of pain, whether it's from bone origin or a true epicondylitis.

Bone disorders come from a variety of sources, including infections where acute/chronic osteomyelitis and TB of bones are mentioned. They are usually associated with systemic complaints of fever, sweating, general malaise and weakness, moderate to severe elbow swelling with increased fluid in the joint. Injuries are accompanied by a history of trauma, falling, accident and/or hitting the elbow on a hard surface. There is normally an obvious crepitating sound and deformity at the elbow. Patients often support the elbow with the normal hand in an attempt to immobilize the injured elbow. Fractures, sublaxations and dislocations are found in this category. Autoimmune conditions often include other general complaints of other joints, polyathritis like in rheumatoid arthritis and a butterfly rash and hair loss in systemic lupus erythromatosus. Bone tumors, though rare, occupying approximately 2% of all tumor types, should be eliminated from the diagnosis. Benign bone tumors are usually localized and can present at the elbow with pain and tenderness, the likes of bone cyst and osteoma. Malignant tumors are possible, but customarily are aggressive. Metastatic bone disease, the spread of cancer to bone from other sites is probable, but the elbow is rarely the secondary site, which is often occupied by the spine, pelvis and chest. Hematological and endocrine disorders can result in bone disease, which are seldom localized. X-rays are the main choice of excluding these states, although some conditions like acute osteomyelitis have a 2-week lag in X-ray presentation. Computer tomograms (CT scans) and Magnetic resonance imaging (MRI) are other important imaging for bone diagnosis differentials. Others include bone biopsy and histopathology, bone aspirates and culture with antibiograms and blood works from routine full blood picture to specialized biochemical substance checks, parathyroid hormone as an example.

c) Joints

A joint is where 2 or more bones come together, like at the elbow. The articulating surfaces are covered by a shiny, white, protective layer, called cartilage. This cartilage allows smooth mobility at the joint. Joints can be damaged by many types of injuries and diseases. Arthritis is considered the wearing of a joint simply by many years of use. This can cause pain, stiffness and swelling. Over time, these joints become severely damaged and disfigured. Arthritis exists of many kinds and has different presentations. Rheumatoid arthritis is an autoimmune disorder, considered the most painful and disabling form of arthritis. The synovial membrane of a joint becomes inflamed, thickened and forms what are known as vegetations or pannus - if seen under a scope they look like seaweed. The articular cartilage is damaged by inflammatory substances, which erode the articulating surface. When cartilage is damaged, it almost always heals with a fibrous cartilage, which is less potent in function than the original cartilage. This disadvantage of cartilage causes further joint damage, as the fibrous tissue interferes with movement. In time the joint becomes fused or ankylosed. Rheumatoid arthritis may affect many joints or only a few. It is a systemic illness with accompanied malaise, muscle atrophy, osteoporosis and changes in vessels, skin, eyes, lungs and heart. Diagnosis is by clinical examination and blood work as well as X-rays. A negative rheumatoid factor does not exclude diagnosis.

Osteoarthritis is another type; unlike rheumatoid arthritis, it is caused by joint degeneration and may manifest from the early 30s. As explained earlier in the book, collagen production decreases with age. Cartilage of joints are formed by type II collagen which changes its quality with time, becoming less effective at its use as a friction protector. Articulating bones rub against each other, causing severe pain and restriction in movement. Osteoarthritic joints may lock, especially of the fingers. Osteoarthritis affects large joints that are used most over a lifetime such as the hip, knee, vertebral column and fingers. X-rays are the mainstay of diagnosis where osteophytes can be seen, and other blood work.

Gout arthritis is an inborn error in metabolism of protein in which a missing enzyme causes the chemical it normally acts on to build up. Uric acid then crystallizes, accumulating in joints to form tophi (lumps of crystals) affecting the elbow and often the big toe. A complete general examination, history and uric acid check in blood together with X-rays are sufficient for diagnosis elimination. Pseudo gout occurs when a different type of crystal other than urates accumulate.

d) Bursa

Bursae are thin slippery sacs, which produce synovial fluid to act as cushions between bones and soft tissues. The olecranon bursa lies between loose skin and the pointy bone at the back of the elbow, the olecranon. Normally the olecranon bursa is flat, but when inflamed it is large, with more fluid production, a condition known as bursitis. Elbow bursitis can occur from trauma, prolonged pressure, infection and disease conditions like gout and rheumatoid arthritis. Main patient complaints include swelling, pain upon bending the elbow, or pressure at times with restricted motion. It may also be accompanied by fever, chills, sweats, and redness around the elbow with breaks in skin- at times discharging pus. Clinical examination with extraction of bursa fluid for laboratory investigations to rule out gout or infection, blood tests, and X-rays may reveal bone spurs.

e) Muscles

The biceps muscle has two heads, the long and short head attach to the humerus and ulna via the tendons and they flex the elbow. The most commn bicep disorders are rupture and tendonitis. Bicep rupture results in a patient being unable to flex the elbow. Bicipital tendonitis occurs in the radial groove where the long head of bicep tendon sits. This, however, is a shoulder complaint with pain, occasional snapping sounds and tenderness, which worsen upon overhead reaching. The triceps muscle, an elbow extensor, may more or less suffer the same fate as that of biceps. Its tendon, when inflamed, causes pain at the back of the elbow, which increases in intensity with stress like punching. Other rare muscle disease conditions such as myositis exist where muscle fibers and skin are inflamed and damaged. Several types are known, some of which are dermatomyositis, polymyositis and inclusion body myositis. Its probability increases in HIV patients and/or people taking antiretroviral drugs, especially zidovudine. General fatigue, muscle weakness and trouble swallowing are some of its presentations. Diagnosis is by electromyography together with nerve induction tests to rule out muscle nerve denervation states.

f) Ligaments

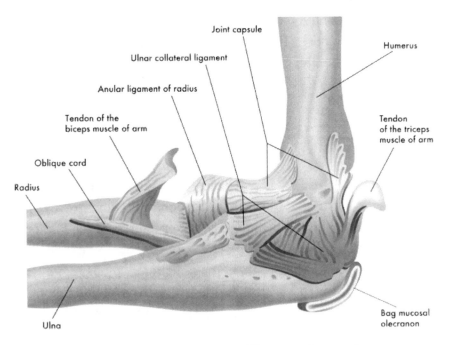

Ligaments are fibrous connective tissue fibers made up of collagen that connects bone to bone. These structures are the key components to a strong joint with stability and strength being their major contribution. Excess strain on the elbow, overstretching and improper exercise techniques can increase weakness and laxity, hence causing instability. Ligament injuries can range from sprains to mild or severe tears, which require surgical intervention.

Ulnar collateral ligaments attach the ulna to the humerus, damage of which causes pain along the medial elbow and can be confused with golfer's elbow. The annular ligament occupies the area around the head of the radius and attaches to the ulna. The little rotational movement possible at the elbow, like opening a door, owes it to this particular anatomy. Injury to the annular ligament causes lateral epicondyle pain and should be differentiated from

26

tennis elbow. Physicians do ligament stress tests on the elbow during physical examination to diagnose it, with MRI as a supporting investigatory imaging.

g) Nerves and vessels in the elbow

Originating from cervical nerve roots, the brachial plexus innervates the upper limb. The main peripheral nerves of the brachial plexus are radial, median and ulnar nerves, which also pass at the elbow joint. Nerve injury in this region is common, especially that of the ulnar nerve. Nerve entrapment syndromes at the elbow have a typical clinical presentation. The ulnar nerve passes behind the medial epicondyle in the ulnar groove and enters the forearm. It travels along the medial part of the forearm to enter the hand at the wrist. Median nerves from the brachial plexus run alongside the brachial artery and descend into the cubital fossa. It gives off branches, which supply the elbow joint. The radial nerve runs posterior to the brachial artery within the triceps muscle. It curves the humeral knob to enter the cubital fossa, running lateral to the forearm to enter the hand. Accompanying theses nerves are blood vessels of the same name. The ulnar artery runs on the anterior and medial side of the elbow while the radial runs anterior and laterally. Both of these arteries are terminal branches of the brachial artery. Brachial, radial and ulnar veins are deeper, though accompany arteries of the same name. You can palpate vessels in the cubital fossa by placing fingers on the anterior of the elbow, feeling the pulse.

At the elbow, pathology of nerves and vessels can occur if they get compressed or directly injured and/or degenerate in some neurovascular disorders such as peripheral neuropathies. A tumor, bony spurs and osteophytes may compress neurovascular bundles at the elbow. If the ulnar nerve is compressed, what is known as the cubital tunnel syndrome, the little finger to half of the ring finger on both the palm and backside become paraesthetic with a tingling sensation. A Tinel sign, tapping at the elbow above the ulnar nerve location can cause these symptoms to reoccur or worsen, thus making the test positive. Nerve conduction studies, X-rays, ultrasound, MRI and clinical examination with trick tests like Tinel sign are adequate to eliminate this diagnosis.

Of difficulty to differentiate is lateral epicondylitis and radial nerve compression at the elbow, as they occur at the same region and may even occur concurrently in the same patient. Radial tunnel syndrome examination may reveal resisted supination and extension, commonly night pain and cramps and sensation loss on the medial surface of forearm. CT scan, MRI and EMGs are helpful.

Elbow median nerve compression is the least occurring, though if it does, is called pronator syndrome. Tinel sign may be positive, with a loss of pinching or picking up a coin using the thumb and index fingers. Also, paraesthesias in the thumb with weakness and atrophy of thenar muscles (a hump of muscles below the thumb on the palmer side) occur. EMGs, MRIs, X-rays and any other investigations in other nerve syndromes described before are required. For vascular conditions such as vasculitis, phlebitis, aneurysm and thromboembolism, angiography is necessary.

h) How can you help your physician arrive at the correct diagnosis?

Physicians can ask a patient extra questions to try and deduce the possible diagnosis and/or candidate conditions. You can assist your physician to make a correct diagnosis of epicondylitis and/or any other which would also mean your recovery time will be reduced as you receive correct treatment to a correct diagnosis. Before attending your doctor's appointment, write down each symptom you are suffering from with a precise description of them without any conclusions. For instance instead of saying "I have epicondylitis," say "I have pain on the side of the elbow." More descriptions of this pain are usually required, such sa describing whether it is a sharp or dull pain or of any other characteristics, localizing it to a specific point or at times to a region. Explain when the pain occurs, whether in the morning, at night or constantly and if it appears during a particular activity, e.g. flexing the elbow. Determine its severity on a scale of 0-10, stating any associations, for instance warmth or redness at the outer elbow. This can be done for every symptom, although knowledge is required on how to describe each complaint, as in specific sub-questions to them. Also jot down any medications that you are taking or have recently been taking, the ones which you feel help in easing your symptoms and those that don't, reporting also any allergic reactions. As an example, ciproflaxin used in treatment of urinary tract infections is a fluoroquinolone. This drug affects tendons and can result in fluoroquinolone-induced tendonitis.

Knowledge of your medical history is essential; by following your family tree and looking at conditions that run through it, one can prevent manifestation of certain hereditary conditions which without a trigger factor do not come to be expressed. Cancer, diabetes and heart disease are some of these hereditary diseases. Epicondylitis can be possible if there is a hereditary collagen defect, which affects connective tissues, but this will usually be more of a diffuse connective tissue disorder and not a single tendon complaint like tennis elbow. If you are planning a trip and/or changing location, it is advised to get an information letter from your previous physician. By law you are entitled to your medical records where only upon asking for authorization for the release of information form can it be possible. This law, however, differs from state to state and country to country. If authorized, a list of what has been done so far, such as tests, X-rays, MRIs, blood work results and medications you have used before, is given to you which you will then show to your new doctor for better treatment.

Chapter 5) Investigations

When your doctor orders investigations or tests such as CT scans
or MRI to differentiate a diagnosis, it is important that you
understand thoroughly why it is required and what the particular
test is about or how it is done. Knowing about a required medical
investigation is good for you because whether invasive or not
medical tests do carry risks associated with their use. It is of
importance that you understand the extent of these risks.

A medical test is a medical procedure done to detect, diagnose or
monitor disease conditions and their processes. There are many
tests that exist and it isn't necessary that you do all of them when
you get ill, but do a few select ones suggested by your physician.
If you are well informed and would want to do a certain test for
whatever reason you may have, you can still suggest it to your
doctor or ask if you can do it.

There are many ways to classify medical tests and still even these
classifications differ from country to country or state to state. By
usage, medical tests are divided into three groups, the first being
diagnostic. Diagnostic tests are performed to confirm a disease
that is already suspected in a patient. For instance, checking blood
sugar levesl in a patient suspected to have diabetes mellitus, or an
electrocardiogram to check heart irregularities in a patient
complaining of chest pain. Then comes another type, a screening
test. It is a procedure done to individuals with a risk of having a
certain medical condition. For example, a Pap smear to screen for
cervical cancer. Other tests can be used for monitoring purposes,
to check the progression of a particular condition. By method,
tests can be as simple as a general physical examination to X-

rays, which are pretty much the basic tests for epicondylitis. An extra classification that does not qualify to be under usage criteria is by location, as such urine tests and blood tests are included.

Truth be told, a wide variety of tests are used in medicine worldwide, some being more famous in other places compared to others due to the fact that disease distributions are different across the globe. If we are to discuss all tests, we can write an over 100-page book on medical investigations alone. In this text we are going to elaborate the main medical tests used in diagnosing epicondylitis and/or its differential diagnosis.

a) X-ray

Radiograph or roentgenograph is a worldwide basic medical test for bone complaints. It is a form of radiation where beams of light, much like radio waves, pass through the region of interest. Dense tissues like bone appear white, since they absorb much of the radiation, soft tissues are grey, and air is black. X-rays are useful in many situations. They are used to detect fractures, dislocations, arthritis, fluid in a joint, bone tumors, bone alignment or its healing after a fracture - these are but a few. This medical test is affordable for many and we can say that it is a standard initial image for bone complaints.

Disadvantages are that X-rays have radiation emission, which can be damaging, especially to body cell-forming organs like the thymus, bone marrow, thyroid, ovaries and testicles, leading to cancer if too much radiation is absorbed. However, this is usually not the case with a single X-ray, but multiple. For instance, exposed radiographers who do X-rays for patients. Pregnancy is a contraindication to this test especially during the first trimester. A lead apron can be used for protection if an X-ray image is really required. At the third trimester, however, it's controversial. The argument is that if X-rays can be done in newborns, why not in a fetus with an already formed skeleton? Nonetheless, lead aprons are the way to go.

b) CT Scan

Computer tomography scan, computed axial tomography (CAT scan), or X-ray computer tomography are all names used to mean the same thing. In a CT scan, an X-ray is processed by a computer to produce cross-sectional images of a specific area of the body. It involves generation of three-dimensional images of the inside of an organ from a series of two-dimensional X-ray images taken around the same axis. CT scans are done by licensed professionals called radiographers. CT scans have a high contrast resolution, which means any differences in density between two tissues by 1% can be distinguished. The quality of resolution on a CT-scan can also be enhanced by the use of a contrast medium. An example of a contrast medium is iodine, which is given intravenously to target a particular organ. The presence of iodine in blood causes greater absorption and scattering of X-ray radiation thus producing a clearer picture of the organ being scanned. CT-scans are often used to image complex fractures, especially around the joints, including the elbow joint because it can reconstruct a particular area in multiple planes. In epicondylitis, due to the fact that a CT scan has more resolution than a basic X-ray image, your physician may require a computer tomography especially for what are called hairline fractures, fractures which involve a crack in a bone, but are not so visible on X-ray imaging.

CAT scans have a downside to their use: since it is ionizing radiation they can directly or indirectly damage DNA in tissues leading to mutations and cancer. 0.4% of all cancers are reported to have occurred in patients, years post CT scans. Kidney problems are another adverse effect of computer tomography associated with reactions to contrast medium.

A CT-scan is produced by a CT gantry machine. A CT gantry machine is a large doughnut-shaped scanner with a table attached to it. During the procedure you lie on the table, and the attached scanner X-rays the part of the body under investigation, slicing the organ thinly with each rotation. All the sliced images are grouped into a single folder and can be printed.

c) MRI

Magnetic resonance imaging (MRI) is a very high-power resolution test, which uses a magnetic field and pulses of radio waves to make pictures of parts of the body under testing, usually soft tissues. MRI is a high-grade test because it can show a problem that cannot be seen with other images, e.g. a torn tendon not shown by ultrasound. Magnetic resonance is done for many reasons. It is used to find many medical conditions or emergencies such as bleeding, vascular disease, infection and cancer. It may be used with contrast substances to produce an even clearer picture. For bones and joints, MRI can check for bone marrow diseases, torn ligaments and tendons, infection, infarction and bone tumors. It is a good choice of test for obese patients.

During the procedure the body is put into a special machine with a strong magnet. Digital images are emitted from the scanner and can be saved on a computer or printed. When the machine is being used one might hear snapping and clicking sounds with air circulating from a fan.

A downside is that people who are claustrophobic may need thorough reassurance and the test may even be substituted. Patients who underwent replacement surgeries such as pacemakers and joint replacements are contraindicated in using this machine since it contains a gigantic magnet - imagining what might happen is in itself scary.

d) Ultrasound

Most of you know what ultrasound is especially if you have had one done before during pregnancy where you could see your unborn baby even at a few weeks. Ultrasound imaging, also called ultrasonography or ultrasound, involves the use of ultrasound gel on the skin to expose the body to high frequency sound waves and using a transducer probe, an internal image can be obtained. The ultrasound machine consists of a computer with a screen for display, electronics and a transducer probe. This probe is a hand-held device, which resembles a microphone, and is attached to the computer by cables. The ultrasound gel helps the transducer to properly contact the skin, eliminating any air pockets between them. The transducer is placed on the elbow joint under testing, moving the probe back and forth until the area is visible on the screen. The probe produces short, non-audible waves which when they hit an object bounce back, being captured by the transducer to reflect an image of the object on the display, its shape, size, and consistency. There is usually no pain, not unless there is some tenderness. This whole procedure takes about 15-30 minutes with immediate results, which can be printed and interpreted by the radiographer.

Unlike X-rays, ultrasound is not ionizing radiation and is very safe, cheap and pain-free. It is a non-invasive procedure, which is used to show structures in real time such as blood flow in vessels and intestine mobility. It can provide reliable images to diagnose tendon and ligament tears, fluid collection in muscles, joints or bursae, and in nerve entrapment conditions such as cubital tunnel syndrome. If one is to have an ultrasound done they should wear comfortable clothes preferably in two pieces so that only the top can be pushed up if an abdominal ultrasound is required, for instance, and in epicondylitis a short-sleeved top will suffice to leave the elbow area free for examination. Ultrasound is very sensitive to motion and this applies especially if children are to be examined, they will need entertainment to keep them still.

Ultrasound is a good replacement for MRI in cases where patients have pacemakers or are claustrophobic and cannot have an MRI done. There are no downsides to its use but some limitations, which include inadequacy to deep tissue examination in obese people and its inability to penetrate bone, making it a soft tissue diagnostic medical imaging.

e) Electromyogram

Muscles are controlled by nerve impulses, which make it react in a particular way. Electromyography is the measurement of electrical activity of muscles at rest and during contractions. This should not be confused with an electromyogram, which can be defined as the waves produced by muscle activity at rest and/or during contraction presented on paper, screen or video. If one is having muscle pain at the elbow or forearm, an EMG can be done to find out how much either the nerve or the muscle is functioning. Per se this checks how your spinal cord nerve roots function. EMGs are done to rule out diseases, which involve muscle weakness, twitching or spasm and those which damage the nerve muscular junction like myasthenia gravis. However, it does not show spinal cord conditions. To prepare for this test, one should avoid stimulants such as caffeine or smoking, and some medications like anticholinergics, which can influence the procedure. An EMG takes about 30-60 minutes to be conducted and involves one being seated in a chair and the forearm under investigation is cleaned. A sterile needle is introduced to the muscle being tested. This needle electrode is connected by wires to a recording machine, which produces waves to show muscle activity at rest. The doctor then asks you to contract the muscle slowly and steadily with subsequent recording of this activity as well. The needle may be moved around in the muscle for good positioning. Pain may be felt as a sharp needle prick, which disappears over 1-2 hours after the procedure. On the screen many spiky waves appear which can be read from the screen or printed. This is done by a doctor or an electromyography specialist. EMG is very safe, though some people may get sore at the needle prick site; infection is rare because sterile needles are used. The EMG results are used along with other medical test results, medical history and physical examination.

f) Nerve conduction test

Nerves control body muscles with electrical signals called impulses. Nerve conduction tests measure impulses as a way of checking the speed of electrical conduction, which can be slow in nerve problems such as cubital syndrome or carpal tunnel syndrome. Nerve conduction tests are therefore used to evaluate the state of the peripheral nervous system.

The nerve conduction procedure involves attaching several flat metal disc electrodes to the skin by tape, then a shock-emitting electrode is placed over the skin lying over the nerve. With a low voltage current, the underlying nerve is excited and the time it takes for the impulse to move from the excited nerve to causing muscle contraction is recorded, what is called conduction velocity. The same procedure can be repeated on the other side for comparison purposes, as it is rare to have the same neurological condition on both sides- unless it's a generalized neurological disease. It takes about 20-60 minutes for the procedure to be carried out. It is important to mention that normal

body temperature should be maintained throughout the procedure
- cold slows down nerve conduction. A conduction nerve test is
carried out prior to the EMG if both tests are required. This
medical diagnostic test is safe, non-invasive, and there are no
downsides to its use except that an uncomfortable muscle twitch
can be felt with each nerve excitation and that some patients may
become anxious.

g) What is blood work?

Blood is composed of two main components, cells and plasma,
where plasma is defined as the liquid portion of blood. Cells such
as red blood cells, white blood cells and platelets float in this
plasma. In the plasma are dissolved substances such as nutrients,
electrolytes, vitamins, hormones and antibodies to fight infection.
The term blood work is a general term used to mean any blood
test that is performed to measure any one of the named blood
components. It could be a test for electrolytes or hormones.
Within these components are sub-components. For instance,
hormones are a vast variety in blood - any specific one can be
picked out, e.g. a test to check for the growth hormone levels in
blood.

After general physical examination with potential candidates for
differential diagnosis in mind, a doctor will order specific blood
work to those candidate conditions. It is thus not necessary to do
each and every blood test that exists. On a different note, blood
can also be cultured to let whatever disease-causing agent in it
grow. This allows diagnosing a particular species of pathogens
and their sensitivity to specific antibiotics can be done
simultaneously. This is of importance in disease conditions such
as bone infection and/or joint infection. A blood test usually
involves a needle attached to a syringe being placed into a blood
vessel - often used is the anterior elbow or wrist. This procedure

takes about 5 minutes and is not particularly painful, but a needle prick is felt as the needle punctures skin and the vein. A sample of blood is drawn and the needle is removed. A cotton swab will be placed at the puncture site and you will be asked to compress to stop the bleeding.

Blood work in epicondylitis is required to differentiate medical conditions such as elbow pain associated with infection, inflammation and/or even a systemic endocrine condition. The tests often used include the likes of C-reactive protein (CRP), erythrocyte sedimentation rate (ESR), full blood picture (FBP), electrolytes such as sodium (Na), potassium (K), Chloride (Cl) and calcium (Ca), hormones inclusive of parathyroid, thyroid and calcitonin. Only a few of these blood tests are going to be discussed due to their close relation to epicondylitis differential diagnosis.

FBP

Full blood picture, also called full blood count (FBC), is by far the most widely used blood test. It is used to assess the general body health of an individual by measuring the cellular component of blood and its subdivisions. The normal cell quantity ranges in blood are known, deviation from which is considered to be a pathology. FBP on its own cannot diagnose a condition, but can give clues and/or support clues. For instance, if epicondylitis is to be differentiated from an elbow infection, on FBP results, white blood cells are expected to be increased in quantity because these cells help the body to fight infection.

ESR

Erythrocyte sedimentation rate is a blood test used to check for the presence of infection or inflammation in the body. It is a simple test done to check how long it takes for a blood drop to move to the bottom of a fluid-filled tube. The longer it takes, the more likely infection/inflammation is to be present. In general, the normal density of a drop of blood in the norm is below 15 millimeters per hour, though variations exist with age. ESR can be used to measure treatment effectiveness, for instance antibiotic effect on an infection. As expected, if the antibiotics are effective the infection decreases until it disappears, as will the ESR. Consecutive tests are done and compared.

CRP

C-reactive protein, sometimes called acute phase protein, is a marker of inflammation/infection. It is produced by the liver as the first substance of response to the presence of inflammation. Like ESR, CRP can be used to monitor treatment efficacy on a particular disease.

Electrolytes

An electrolyte test, also known as an electrolyte balance test, is used to measure different kinds of electrolytes in blood. Electrolytes play many roles in the blood circulatory system where excretion of waste products, stabilizing acidity and alkalinity and metabolism are mentioned. Sodium (Na), potassium (K), and chloride (Cl) are the most often checked, since they are the three main electrolytes in the body, but depending on the system under investigation other electrolytes can be added, for instance calcium (Ca) in bone diseases.

Blood culture

A blood culture involves taking a small sample of blood from your vein. This blood is laced in a medium with nutrients and left to 'grow,' bacterial growth known as culturing. The idea is that even if there are traces of bacteria in the blood, growing them will multiply them to a level where it will be possible to detect them.

Chapter 6) Tennis Elbow

Is this the kind of pain you are experiencing?

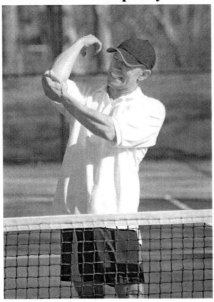

a) Is tennis elbow inflammation or a torn tendon? What exactly is it?

The term tennis elbow has been used since 1883 when Major used it in his paper "Lawn-tennis elbow." This is actually a misnomer since only 5% of all tennis elbow cases have actually developed from playing tennis. Well, tennis elbow is neither inflammation nor a torn tendon, but for a better understanding, we can compare a heart infarct, which is instant and precise to atherosclerosis, cholesterol plaque accumulation in vessels over a lifetime. Tennis elbow is more of the atherosclerosis type, slow, degenerative and occurring over a long period of time until a certain endpoint is reached when symptoms first appear. We can say it is tendinosis. Flare-ups or exacerbation episodes may occur and can present with a heart infarct type of picture. This does not necessarily mean that the condition has worsened and/or the tendon has ruptured, but just an increased aggravation of the symptoms after maybe a long tennis game and/or long drive. Flares often are recognized as flares because symptoms often exist in a mild or moderate form prior to their occurring. You would have known if it were an acute injury: it often swells, becoming warm and red.

Tennis elbow starts out gradually, with no symptoms until a certain threshold of tendon injury occurs, where pain at the lateral epicondyle appears as the first symptom. This means that long before symptoms appear, the extensor carpi radialis brevis muscle tendon fibers have been building up tension, with destruction of a few fiber lengths at a particular time. Then, over time, the quantity of injured fibers pass a threshold mark, irritating the nerve endings, thus being perceived as pain.

For many years, tendonitis has been blamed for tennis elbow, though research has for decades proven otherwise. It must be the drug companies who do not want you to know this. It is difficult at times to break such traditions, in this case the notion that tendonitis is the primary causative devil of lateral epicondylitis. If we understand what inflammation is, maybe many will realize that it was but a scam by the initial theory deducers.

Therefore, what is inflammation?

The term inflammation comes from the Latin word "inflammo" meaning ignite or set alight. It is a normal body response to harmful stimuli, set as an attempt to self-protect. Inflammation is a protective mechanism against disease-causing agents, chemical substances and damaged cells, and it is the initial phase in the healing process. Infection and inflammation are two different processes where infection is caused by pathogens such as viruses, bacteria or fungus, while inflammation is the body's response to it. The immune system includes inflammation as one of its components where it constitutes our innate immunity. Innate immunity is inborn body protection. Even though inflammation is a good guy, it can be a robber, since inflammation can cause further inflammation, a too-much-can-be-harmful sort of thing. This fundamental pathological process consists of dynamic, complex, microscopic, apparent cytological changes, with infiltration and mediator release that occurs in affected or injured tissues. Naked to the eye, its presence can be noted by the so-called cardinal signs of inflammation. These are pointer symptoms for one to conclude that, yes, inflammation is present as such redness, warmth, swelling, pain and loss or inhibited function are named. Some of these signs may be seen in certain conditions, but none are necessarily present at once. Inflammation can be further divided into acute or chronic, acute being of rapid onset with a quick change to become severe. Symptoms are present for a few days and may persist to a few weeks. Sore throat from a flu, acute appendicitis and acute tonsillitis are examples of disease conditions that can result in acute inflammation. Chronic inflammation refers to long–term, lasting for several months to years, and can result as a complication of acute inflammation, failure of the body to overpower the stimulus causing it and/or a persistent low intensity stimulus. Asthma, rheumatoid arthritis, chronic peptic ulcer disease and tuberculosis are examples.

With that said, whether or not your physician says you have tennis elbow or tendonitis, lateral epicondylitis diagnosis is almost always based on the simple description of your symptoms.

b) Causes

Myth has it that tennis elbow affects only tennis players. This is not so, because 95% of all reported cases are from non-tennis players. Tennis elbow is primarily caused by overuse at the elbow joint and it can affect anyone. Any repetitive elbow movements such as gardening, painting with rollers, plumbing or using hand tools can cause tennis elbow, even simple activities like screw driving. In short, any activity that requires constant elbow flexion and extension or excessive use of forearm and hand muscles can result in this condition appearing. Some tennis playing techniques are great contributors to lateral epiconylitis development. The following are listed:

a) Hitting the ball too late during the backhand

b) Extending the wrist on a follow-through

c) A new racket with taut strings and a very large handle

d) One-handed backstrokes

e) Leading a hit with the elbow instead of the racket

f) Oversized racket heads, though, have a larger surface area to prevent mishits, increase vibration forces.

g) Lightweight rackets, designed to allow older groups to play at the expense of overstraining the elbow, especially if opponent is a big server.

h) Rough court surfaces

i) Faulty technique, i.e. hitting the ball in a biomechanically unsafe position.

Other individual-specific risk factors consist of poor flexibility, disease conditions such as spondylosis of the back, biceps insufficiency, frozen shoulder and age groups over thirty.

Sporting activities dependent on elbow activity are listed, baseball, basketball, squash, table tennis, softball to mention but a few.

c) Symptoms

Excess amounts of monotonous or quick motions that involve eccentric contractions (contraction of a muscle as it lengthens), gripping of forearm muscles can lend you a tennis elbow. Main symptoms of lateral epicondylitis include pain and tenderness, loss of strength, stiffness and swelling. The pain is felt on the lateral side of the elbow and the top of the forearm. It is usually a dull ache felt when the elbow is active, subsiding with rest. This is the early sign of the diagnosis upon which if ignored can worsen to become more intense and frequent, if not constant even at rest. A burning sensation may accompany the pain, radiating to the wrist and hand. Tennis elbow affects the arm you use the most, right for right-handers with left following suit. As the condition progresses, holding items and carrying loads becomes difficult, even a task like lifting a mug of coffee. Muscle weakness accompanied by tingling and numbness may be felt in the forearm or hand. The joint becomes hard to move, feeling stiff and resistant. If left untreated, it can permanently lead to a contracture with inability to bend or straighten the elbow.

d) Diagnosis

Tennis elbow diagnosis is always based on its classical clinical picture, that are symptoms and signs. A physician will examine the elbow in such a way that the tennis elbow diagnosis is confirmed by the end of the routine elbow examination, if it actually is and/or a list of all differentials. See, feel, and move is the examination triad recommended by Apley, which is widely used by orthopaedic specialists. At "see," the physician looks at the elbow skin from all directions in search for scars, whether they resulted from injury or previous surgery. Under observation is also the skin texture, noting any disorders such as vascular scars, psoriasis and any swellings. "Feel" follows and a physician touches the elbow surface to check for temperature, comparing it to other regions of the limb for warmth or heat, which are easily appreciated during this process. Any swelling is felt between the thumb and index finger for mobility and consistency. Any cysts are usually fluid-filled and lipomas thick-textured. In addition, feeling localizes the point or region of pain depending on whether a localized point like the lateral epicondyle is affected or diffuse wider area at the elbow region. The final examination stage of the elbow is crucial to appreciate the extent of any functional loss. The degree of flexion, extension, pronation and supination flexibility is measured, deficit of which can greatly compromise elbow movement. It is not only general random movements that are checked, but also tricky movements with purpose known as tests or signs. For instance, Cozen's test, also called resistance tennis elbow test, is performed with the elbow in extension. The patient then extends the wrist against resistance by the physician triggering pain on the lateral aspect of the elbow owing to stress applied over the extensor carpi radialis brevis tendon. Mill's test is also performed as a passive test. The examiner passively pronates the patient's forearm, followed by wrist flexion. Any pain felt on the lateral elbow constitutes a positive test. Other tests include the chair lifting test and Maudsley's test. Chair lifting test employs the individual under examination to lift the back of a chair using 3 fingers (thumb, index and middle finger) with an extended elbow. Any lateral epicondyle pain expresses a positive. In Maudsley's, the third finger is extended under resistance, exciting pain on a positive test.

As discussed in prior chapters, differential diagnosis is a must. Moreover, the elbow stability substances also have their specific tests. Ligament stability tests, the valgus and varus test, are carried out. In valgus, the examiner fixes the elbow with the left hand if right–handed, and vice versa if left–handed, soon after which an outward movement of the forearm at the elbow joint is applied. Any abnormal displacement of the articulating bones show a medial (ulnar) collateral ligament sprain. Repeating this whole procedure, but with inward varus stress, shows lateral (radial) collateral ligament instability if the test is positive. The elbow flexion test, where a patient maximally flexes the elbow, holding the position for 3-5 minutes, is a nerve compression test. Radiating pain along the median nerve distribution is positive for cubital fossa syndrome.

Previously discussed Tinel's sign is also another test often done. There are just so many of these which specialists such as an orthopaedic surgeon, sports medicine specialist and physiotherapist use on a daily basis and as such are the right people to see where tennis elbow diagnosis is suspected.

Blood tests and imaging investigations are not to be forgotten. X-rays are the most frequently ordered by physicians and are considered to be basic as they are affordable to most, if not all, patients. Specialized imaging such as MRI and CT scan are very expensive for both the patient and provider, which is why they are used by a physician only if necessary. All these efforts to arrive at a tennis elbow diagnosis are usually sufficient.

e) Treatment

In previous chapters we learned how to recognize tennis elbow and to differentiate it from other disease conditions. Millions of players are kept from playing tennis by lateral epicondylitis. Perhaps you have witnessed elbow braces on players struggling to keep playing despite their sore elbow. Tennis elbow is a self-limiting condition, which means that it can eventually get better without treatment, yet may still last several weeks or months. Strength of a unit area of a tendon is comparable to that of bone and as such tendons heal slowly. Though tennis elbow treatment is often successful, surgery is a last resort if other treatments aren't helpful.

Treatment modalities are individually specific and are determined by your consultant or physiotherapist based on age, medical history, general health, severity of condition, tolerance to medications, procedures and therapies, expectation of the course of the condition and your opinion or preference. However, as the myth goes, a doctor is the only one who can cure your tennis elbow. Once the correct diagnosis has been made, one can easily follow step-by-step pain relief programs at home. By law it is a patient's right to accept, deny or opt for particular treatment plans once completely informed.

Treatment plans of tennis elbow are divided into two broad groups, namely conservative and surgical intervention.

Conservative treatment includes:

a) Avoiding the activity that produces the symptoms. Avoiding the causative activity is of great importance, without which chronic symptoms may persist for months and years with no relief.

b) Pharmacological symptomatic treatment can be used, where typically non-steroidal anti-inflammatory drugs (NSAIDs) are used to relieve pain, though they do not contribute to the overall functional outcome. NSAIDs often used are ibuprofen, diclofenac and naproxen, which can be used as oral tablets, topical gels and/or injections. They are effective for short-term pain relief. NSAIDs are a class of pharmacological drugs that provide anti-pain, antipyretic and anti-inflammatory effects all in one and are not recommended during pregnancy, in particular the third trimester. NSAIDs are not directly teratogenic, but are linked to miscarriages and premature birth. Knowledge of their adverse effects is essential, especially during prolonged use or at high doses among which headache, dizziness, constipation, nausea, diarrhea, excess gas, extreme weakness and fatigue are listed. It is contraindicated for use in patients with peptic ulcer disease and other gastrointestinal medical conditions. Simultaneous use of proton pump inhibitors like omeprazole or rabeprazole is protective against these negative effects. Other medications like acetaminophen (Tylenol) are effective substitutes. Do not be carried in the myth bandwagon that states that drugs can cure epicondylitis. That myth has long been busted, as pain medicines temporarily relieve pain; once they wear off, the pain begins again.

c) Modifying tennis playing choices
Racket selection can be difficult, although if you understand their mechanical faults, choosing one with tennis elbow protection in mind will be easy. Racket weight and balance have a great effect on deducing how much potentially harmful force from a racket ball impact is transferred to your arm. More weight of the racket is relatively safe, better still if most of it is localized at the head. 11 ounces is recommended, which provides more shock-absorbing capacity and torsion force resistance. Looser, thinner

and more resilient strings are perfect for painful elbow prevention. The peak shock transferred to the forearm from ball impact is delayed and significantly reduced by stretch. A flexible racket frame is generally favorable, though vibrations occurring after ball-on-racket impact are uncomfortable to most players, thus they counter that by tying strings more tightly or using greater force, increasing the probability of lateral epicondylitis. Racket over-gripping is a plus for both your elbow and racket. Smaller-sized tend to break when they accidentally fall on the court, especially a hard court after slipping.

Tennis ball choices do matter. Standardized sizes are 56-59 grams, though can change weight, for instance when wet. This considerably heavier version increases stress to the forearm muscles. In Asia, famous soft tennis as well can be enjoyable. The balls weigh 30-32 grams, which is by far light and sparing to the elbow. Intermediate sizes of 45 grams often used by juniors can be fun for all age groups only if players know what's at stake. Court qualities determine your physique in the game, speed, ball bouncing with an ultimate effect on your legs and hence your biomechanical position. A hard court allows for fast ball rolling, which may be quite brutal to the arm, especially for first-timers. Clay is considered easy on the elbow, though not predictable, with grass considered the worst. Body position in space on the courtyard and during hitting the ball is another risk factor that can be modified. Leg position upon swinging fully and meeting the ball in front allows the body thrust to assist in pushing the ball forward, reducing strength used at the elbow. Do not generate power with the small muscles of your arm. Create power by using big muscles and the kinetic chain to transfer the power to the racket. "Easy power" though, will not fully protect you from tennis elbow. Some professional players can still get lateral epicondylitis by spending the day practicing one-handed backhand top-spin lobs (even when using the correct one-handed backhand top-spin lob technique). Overuse is still the enemy. Protective bracing or plastering of the elbow is often used by most players to put some weight off a strained tendon. Off-court watchfulness is also necessary, especially during typing and sleeping in the proper position and posture should be maintained.

d) Corticosteroid injections are sometimes used to treat particularly painful musculoskeletal problems of which tennis elbow is one of them. Corticosteroids are a type of medication that contain manmade versions of cortisol, a hormone found in humans. In a lifetime, about a maximum of three injections are allowed, above which they become harmful. However, clinical evidence revealed that their use for tennis elbow treatment is limited. The injection is given directly at the painful point on the elbow side, usually after numbing the area with local anaesthetic. Cortisone is the widely used drug. Long-term use of corticosteroids can bring about severe adverse effects such as menstrual problems, weight gain, irregular heartbeat, flashes, changes in vision, steroid-induced diabetes, osteoporosis and peptic ulcer disease. Therefore, prolonged oral use is generally not recommended unless deemed otherwise by your physician, who prescribes the doses with tapering techniques.

e) Autologous blood injection (ABI) and platelet-rich plasma injection (PRP) can be used. ABI involves injecting a patient's own blood into a damaged tendon. This method uses knowledge that blood contains a lot of cells and growth factors required for healing. The difference between ABI and PRP is that in PRP only blood plasma is used. Blood is extracted from a vein, then is centrifuged to harvest plasma which then is used for injecting into the tendon. Platelets are small fragment cells, which aggregate during the process of blood clotting. These platelets contain platelet-derived growth factors (PDGF), which are essential for growth and tissue regeneration. These injections are given once, after which if there is no relief a repeated dose can be given. Rarely can a patient be injected three times; if there is no relief after two injections, alternative treatment options are used. It is known to be effective with 80% of patients responding well with complete pain relief and/or recovery.

f) Botulinum toxin A (Botox) injected into muscles of the forearm has also been shown to be effective in tennis elbow treatment. It is usually used in severe forms, in which surgery is considered without an immediate tendon continuity disruption. Botox causes temporary muscle paralysis at site of injection, which allows tendon healing. A study done in Hong Kong has proven that pain scores decrease in 4-12 weeks in a random controlled trial with normal saline. However, a second study did not show any improvement of pain, grip strength and quality of life after 12 weeks. Further studies are thus required before Botox can be recommended as treatment of tennis/golfer's elbow.

g) Splinting is also widely used as it provides compression at the elbow, which relieves pain. Splints of many kinds exist and they are going to be explained in detail in further chapters of the book. It is necessary to inform that splints should not be immobilizing, but compressing - the former leads to worsening joint function and may result with a fixed position of the joint, thus completely losing function. Scientifically, they have not been shown to help with pain or recovery of tennis elbow.

h) Ongoing treatment options include exercise and physical therapy treatments to decrease pain and to improve function by maintaining range of motion. More on detailed physiotherapy is explained under the physiotherapy chapter, although it's necessary to mention that before following a certain exercise routine it is important to consult with an expert to see whether you need to change how you do an activity or what equipment to use. A sports trainer, physiotherapist, occupational therapist and ergonomic specialist are the right people for this task.

i) Ultrasound therapy (Orthrotripsy) may help heal your tendon and stop pain, same as shockwave therapy. Shockwave therapy (lithotripsy) is a non-invasive treatment where high-energy shockwaves are passed through the skin. Minor side effects include bruising and reddening of the skin in the area being treated, so the risk of treatment trial in a possible burn result is usually not worth it.

j) Magnetic therapy if used in the correct way may be an efficient treatment for epicondylitis. Application of this low-frequency magnetic therapy is thought to relax muscles, improve blood circulation and speed up tendon metabolism. Magnetic therapy is known to reduce pain much better than ice. Two types of magnetic therapy elbow products are available, the first kind being a form of magnetic therapy with far infrared therapy combination. This kind is really heavy. The second type is similar to the usual sports elbow wrap. It is made from stretchable material such as spandex or neoprene. It consists of only far infrared therapy. Scientists believe that tissues and cells give off electromagnetic impulses and that disease arises when these impulses are disrupted. Magnetic therapy is based on an attempt to restore this electromagnetic balance. The procedure of magnetic therapy involves placing static magnets of various sizes and strength onto the affected area. Static magnets have a constant magnetic field, whereas electromagnets have a magnetic field only when electricity is passing through them. Negative magnetic therapy is said to increase tissue oxygen consumption and reduce tissue acidity, therefore supporting metabolism, which is required in the healing of any body tissue. Depending on the disease being treated, therapy can be given for a few minutes to several days. Research studies supporting the effectiveness of magnetic therapy in epicondylitis treatment are scant. It seems like it's more theory than practical. By 2012 the FDA had not approved marketing of magnets for health benefits, but they considered them safe for use except in pregnant women and patients with metallic implants. More research on this subject is called for.

k) Rest, Ice, Compression and Elevation, the so-called RICE method, is a famous symptomatic therapy regimen often used in muscle injuries, though often understood by physicians for its use after an acute injury. Its use on tennis elbow is controversial if not condition-worsening. Nonetheless, at acute or initial stage of tennis elbow many sufferers claim relief. Let's go through the RICE principle:

Rest - this does not mean that one becomes bedridden, but temporarily avoiding or stopping all activities that potentially worsen your injury. Keeping the elbow mobile to restore range of movement and blood flow will aid the healing process.

Ice - never put ice directly on skin as this may lead to thermal skin damage, but preferably use an ice pack wrapped in a towel or cloth. A bag of frozen peas for an unknown reason is somehow famous and works as well as an ice pack. Apply for 10-20 minutes, stopping when the area numbs.

Compression - by using a bandage or wrap over the ice pack. Do not at any point wrap it too tightly as it will cause tissue hypoxia by cutting off blood supply.

Elevate - raise the elbow above the heart level, place it on an arm rest or mount of pillows. This decreases swelling in the elbow as there is less blood pooling.

RICE is recommended every 4-6 hours for up to 48 hours after injury. If there is no relief within 48 hours, consult your physician for examination and diagnosis with initiation of a correct treatment plan. If relief is felt with RICE, increase strength and endurance in tendons, ligaments and muscles around the elbow.

l) Active Release Technique (ART) works on the principle that an injured elbow with time develops adhesions and scar fibrous tissues, which cause pain because they restrict movement. In this treatment plan, these adhesions are released by manipulated stretch of the joint under anaesthesia, followed by physiotherapy to maintain the newly acquired mobility. If inadequate post-adhesion release physio is done, even more adhesions form, contracting the elbow more than before.

m) Prolotherapy is a process of injecting an irritative substance, such as glucose, directly into the injured tendon with the aim of causing temporary swelling, triggering a more pronounced healing response. Unlike corticosteroids, which temporarily reduce pain, but allow disease course to continue, prolotherapy helps total injury healing and recurrence by causing tightening and thickening of the tendon, after which physiotherapy is implemented gradually to achieve the lost full range of motion and/or maintain it.

Sufferers of tennis elbow are individuals with their own particular lifestyles. Natural therapy is yet another option. Natural regimens for tennis elbow treatment are also effective. Besides the RICE method, there's acupuncture, nutrition, herbal medicine, homoeopathy, salts and exercises (see chapter on physiotherapy). Acupuncture is popular and involves the use of fine needles in order to correct qi or energy flow in the body. Many people report relaxation and significantly longer pain relief. If needles sound scary, opt for laser acupuncture. Nutrition uses for tennis elbow treatment can be helpful. Supplementing vitamins and elements is their mainstay. Vitamin C is required for cellular growth and repair. Vitamin E, an antioxidant, destroys free radicals that are released by inflammation. Vitamin A in the form of beta-carotene is needed for collagen synthesis. Combining supplements, for instance, zinc, together with vitamin A, or selenium and vitamin E limits inflammation and speeds up healing. Foods that are used commonly in Asia to reduce swelling and inflammation are turmeric and cumin. Herbal medicines include fenugreek, St. John's wort and curcumin. Homoeopathy is treatment of an illness based on tracing disease symptom patterns and considering how a patient is as an individual. It is known to work best when tennis elbow is acute, Ruta and Rhus tox being the most famous. Silicea and Ferrum phos salts help tennis elbow of a slow healing kind.

Nevertheless, the good news is that in as many as 9 out of 10 people who have tennis elbow, their symptoms disappear and people can actually become carefree and active whether conservative or surgical treatment was used. The main concepts of correct treatment are 5 phases, being pain reduction, inflammation reduction, healing induction, fitness maintenance and controlling the force applied on injured tissues after a correct diagnosis. Physiotherapy is, however, also necessary to maintain full range of motion and to maintain alignment.

Surgery is considered as a last resort when all conservative treatments fail. Indications to surgery include an acute injury that left larger tears in the tendon or severe elbow damage with more than 6 months of tendon rest and rehab with no relief. Many surgical operating techniques exist, where skill is dependent upon the surgeon's experience. Different versions of the surgery can be done, but of the same type of procedure, for instance percutaneous, arthroscopic and/or open surgery versions exist.

Ossatripsy, a process of cutting the tendon from the lateral epicondyle, is done. Lithotripsy can be used concomitantly to protect the damaged area from reinjuring. The arm is then immobilized in a cast or sling with elevation to keep swelling at a minimum. Tennis elbow surgery does not require one to be admitted; it often is done as an outpatient procedure. After surgery, it takes about 4 weeks to determine the surgery's success. Early use of the arm can result in permanent elbow damage.

With any surgery there are risks associated with anaesthesia, excess bleeding, infection and possible iatrogenic nerve damage. The arm can become worse in comparison to its state before surgery. Surgery is no guarantee that you will be pain–free, although a lot of evidence is in our support as a few complicated cases have been reported with a high effectiveness rate. Nonetheless, a thorough surgical risk consideration is prompted before you decide to go under the knife, making sure you have well researched references of the best orthopaedic specialists in town.

f) Prognosis and cure

Whether a cure for tennis elbow exists or not is a mystery. On the other hand, medical evidence supports the notion that it does, though it depends on how you look at it. The American Association for Orthopaedic Surgeons (AAOS) reported that 80-95% of tennis elbow can be successfully treated without surgery and 80-90% of those operated upon. If we calculate approximations of the remaining 5-20% in whom the condition progresses without surgery and 10-20% after surgery, if postulated to the population in question of all patients of lateral epicondylitis, you will notice that the numbers of failed treatment are actually large, thus building controversies towards the notion. However, initial tennis elbow therapy in most cases is adequate to elicit remission, but relapses occur at 18-50%. In most cases 40% of all sufferers have prolonged moderate discomfort.

Age groups divide outcome with 42% of over 50 years suffering severe forms and/or disability, in comparison to about 24% in those below. Women have, however, more symptoms than men, but occurrence of the disease stands at a 1:1 ratio. Nevertheless, other literature reports that men have a marginally higher general prevalence rate, though it was found to be statistically insignificant. The bottom line is that with proper treatment, tennis elbow symptoms can be kept at bay and/or completely eliminated.

Chapter 7) Golfer's Elbow

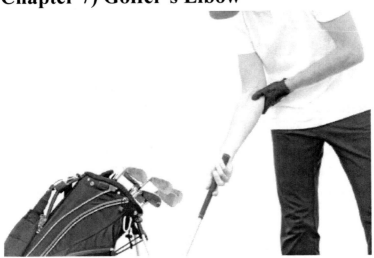

a) What is it?

Medial epicondylitis is commonly known as golfer's elbow. As we mentioned before, it does not occur only in golfers, though poor golf swing techniques contribute to its development and progression. Other repetitive activities, such as operating a chain saw, meat cutters and hand tools result in overuse of muscle tendons at their origin point at the medial epicondyle, leading to golfer's elbow. Like tennis elbow, golfer's elbow is tendinosis with a combination of tendonitis. However, tennis elbow occurs approximately ten times more. Tennis and golfer's elbow are very similar in that they both are overuse medical conditions, though they differ in pain location at the elbow and activities that cause them.

b) Causes

The mechanism of golfer's elbow injury can vary from an acute violent action to most commonly RSIs (repetitive strain injuries) where an activity is performed over and over again until a failure point is reached. Failure point will be known by the development of symptoms, in particular pain and tenderness localized on the inside of the elbow. Just because we have come to know that playing golf is not the main cause does not mean it isn't true. Playing golf with the below listed techniques can provide a risk platform for the development of golfer's elbow:

a) Playing golf without warm-up exercises to the shoulders, elbow, back, hips and legs
b) Dehydration and poor rehydration as the game commences
c) Not being aware of the environment, especially other players and golf balls.
d) Powering up a swing through water
e) Wrong sized golf clubs and grip
f) Poor swing mechanics
g) Too heavy and unbalanced equipment

Some of you might look back and wonder, "But I never do those." Well, there are many other relative factors involved. As mentioned under tennis elbow, genetics, concomitant medical diseases such as diabetes, obesity and hypertension are poor prognosis enhancers. It isn't like a lottery where a single person from millions is picked out. There have to be factors that lead to – well, you know the rest of the story. Finding that particular risk factor is your journey to eliminating golfer's elbow. It is, however, unfortunate to state that not everyone can deduce these factors until a physician or sports trainer evaluates your symptoms and techniques.

c) Pathophysiology

Nirschl proposed four stages to describe epicondylar tendinosis. This staging applies to both medial and lateral epicondylitis with an outline as follows:

Stage 1: exhibits the general inflammatory process within the tendon.

Stage 2: injury is characterized by pathologic tissue alterations. In an effort to repair, fibroblasts produce collagen molecules of type III instead of the usual type I, resulting in a less efficient building material, which is bound to degenerate in the presence of RSIs.

Stage 3: structural failure is the hallmark of this stage.

Stage 4: even with repetitive micro-tears and injury, the tendon continues to repair in an effort to return to its original state with repetition of stages 2 and 3 over and over till a bulk fibrous tissue scar forms, which at times has calcifications.

The final product yielded after stage 4 is an abnormal version of the true tendon, altering typical biomechanics of the elbow.

d) Symptoms

Golfer's elbow in many decades has drawn less attention in relation to tennis elbow, hence there exists far less literature regarding its existence, maybe also due to the fact that its frequent incidence is at 10-20% of all diagnosed epicondylitis. In golfer's elbow the common flexor tendon originating on the medial bony prominence of the elbow is stretched during the acceleration phase of throwing and swinging. The pronator teres and flexor carpi radialis muscles are the most afflicted muscles in this condition. Yet again, as in tennis elbow, symptoms often develop gradually as a dull ache on the medial epicondyle appearing only during activity. Late or no treatment allows the condition to progress to a more intense, severe, symptomatic picture observed during activity and/or even at rest. Pain and tenderness are seen to be the main consistent chief complaints in most sufferers. Radiation of pain down the medial forearm surface into the wrist and hand is uncommon. Swelling and warmth can also be appreciated during examination.

Other differential conditions are also eliminated using the order described under tennis elbow. Of importance to mention is that Dr. Nirschl, an expert on golfer's and tennis elbow, has done a lot of research on tendon injuries, and he divided the medial epicondyle into three zones for the sole purpose of ulnar nerve differential diagnosis. The first zone is the area proximal to the medial epicondyle, the second being at the medial epicondyle itself and third zone distal to it. The zones have been shown to be useful in golfer's elbow sufferers with concomitant ulnar nerve compression. Zone three was proven by Nirschl in individuals who underwent golfer's elbow surgery to be the most common site of compression.

e) Diagnosis

Your physician will take a detailed medical history. He/she will ask you to answer some questions about your pain, how it affects your daily activities, what activity or medication relieves or aggravates it, any past medical injuries to the elbow. Physical examination is the gold mine to diagnosing golfer's elbow. Using the see, feel, and move technique described in chapter 5 with additions of specific golfer's elbow tests, a physician can arrive at the golfer's elbow diagnosis and/or candidate conditions to your complaints. 2 main specific golfer's tests exist and are just called golfer's elbow tests. In one, the patient makes a fist using the involved limb, the examiner then palpates along the medial epicondyle with one hand, and with the other grasps the patient's wrist and passively supinates the forearm extending the elbow, wrist and fingers. Discomfort felt along the medial elbow side marks a positive test. In the second golfer's elbow test, the forearm is pronated in palm-up position, pronated pose with simultaneous wrist flexion at the same time twisting the elbow to face the palm down and wrist towards them. Pain on the medial epicondyle represents yet again a positive test. On the website pthaven.com these tests can be appreciated on video.

Investigations as always are performed, basic blood work and X-rays. Specific tests such as MRI and ulnar nerve conduction tests can also be checked if required. Cubital nerve syndrome is very much similar to golfer's elbow and an experienced physician will know better than to exclude it from the diagnosis.

f) Treatment

Treatment modalities of epicondylitis share the same concept, whether it's medial or lateral. Many approaches to treatment plans exist and differ from specialist to specialist, but in general are a juggle of all the kinds of treatment explained in chapter 5. Choice of treatment is usually made on an individual basis, which is why it's important for you to see a specialist for correct diagnosis and treatment.

After a general sweep through the Internet, praise is being sung to exercise by most sufferers, with many changing this treatment to that or combining the different modes in search of a savior. Will it be harsh to say it's more of a trial and error thing even though eventually every sufferer finds a treatment they call their own? Treatment controversies among users can be discouraging, especially if they are told by an influential individual. The epicondylitis treatment approach I prefer is the three-phase therapy.

Phase 1 - One myth that requires busting is that a sufferer has to stop doing their favorite hobby completely or put their career on hold - wrong. One can still continue with normal activities, though the key point is that one has to make sure that in the process, they are implementing proven tennis elbow or golfer's elbow treatment programs. In severe cases it may still be required to temporarily stop activities that aggravate pain and other symptoms. Total inactivity, however, is not recommended. The biomechanics of a joint, ligament and/or tendon is such that continuous activity is maintained if function is to be preserved, without which muscles waste and atrophy, ligaments and tendons contract, forming fibrotic adhesions, which fix the joint to a permanent contracture. This will totally compromise any rehabilitative efforts. Daily 15 to 20 minutes of icing intervals are done, 3-4 times a day. Controversies suggest that heat works better than cold since heating causes dilatation of blood vessels, allowing more blood to flow to the joint. Accompanying the increase in blood flow are growth factors, cells and nutrients necessary for healing. Others even suggest a combination of both ice and heat where before exercise one ices the elbow, with heat application at the end of the session. Oral non-steroidal anti-inflammatory drugs may be given for 1-2 weeks if patient has no known contraindications to the medication. If symptoms reduce, but are not completely eliminated, the dose can be prolonged to over 2 weeks. Many people argue the fact that pain is a mechanism in which the body responds to injury, like an alarm signal to notify you that something is wrong somewhere. If this pain is eliminated by medication, then one will never know if they have been injured, leading to progression of epicondylitis to a critical nonreversible stage, like in a Charcot joint. But then again, it is unethical to knowingly cause pain.

If none of these measures elicit relief, splinting at night and corticosteroid injection are introduced. Many sufferers I have encountered reported that night splinting alone was a waste, relief was only felt when they started splinting 24/7, making sure the support was not put on too tightly. Besides the fact that this is usually not recommended, it's strange, however, that the forbidden is actually serving many. Shockwave and ultrasound are other alternatives at this phase at doses of 10 minutes approximately 5 times in a fortnight.

Phase 2 begins when one of the phase 1 treatment plans has eliminated the acute epicondylitis symptoms of pain, tenderness, swelling and warmth. A guided rehabilitation program is the hallmark of this phase. Rehabilitation means to restore to good capacity or condition and may prove to be costly, though effective. The first goal of rehabilitation is to achieve full range of motion in the elbow, i.e. flexion, extension, supination and pronation followed by isometric exercises. As flexibility and total range movement returns, resistive exercises are added together with the expected strength. The ultimate goal at this point is to achieve tendon strength equivalent to that of pre-injury or better. As soon as the patient can perform all required tasks without any signs of discomfort, they are introduced back to sport or to the activity that stimulated epicondylitis development in the first place. Rehabilitation does not only cover the injured muscle tendons, but a general musculature sharpening is done for optimal flexibility and stamina.

Phase 3 is closure to a once existing condition and preventing against relapses. Under a personal trainer or coach, a patient's technique is monitored and corrected if required, with attention to equipment choice, i.e. golf clubs of the correct size, weight and grip. Physician's monitoring is also still required though the patient is disease-free. Maintenance of general body flexibility, strength and endurance is a must.

Surgical treatment is the choice of treatment for all acutely torn tendons where a break in continuity is visible on MRI; these injuries have a poor prognosis if treated conservatively. Surgery is also the best choice for all chronic cases with more than 3 months of noninvasive treatment with no improvement. Due to the proximity of the ulnar nerve to the medial epicondyle, open surgery is always recommended. A surgeon will expose and transpose the nerve before any manipulations to prevent its injury. Thus, percutaneous or arthroscopic surgery on golfer's elbow requires high specialization. Mainstay of surgical treatment for golfer's elbow involves tendon debridement and/or release. The tendon is detached from the medial epicondyle, excising any injured portions, then reattaching it firmly to its origin, correcting any local defects, ultimately repositioning the ulnar nerve if it is compressed.

g) Post-operative care

Days 1-3: wound dressing is applied after surgery and this dressing needs to be kept clean and dry, elevating the arm on a pillow or sling to reduce swelling. Analgesics are used before the anesthesia wears off and continued as required after that.

Days 3-14: the wound is kept clean and dry with removal of the post-surgery dressing. Exercise of joints should continue avoiding heavy use of the arm and/or dangling it down at the wrist. Light activity is, however, recommended.

2 weeks: stitches should be removed 10-14 days post-surgery, continue physiotherapy where isometric exercises commence. If wound is completely healed, massage with cream to prevent scarring.

6 weeks: activities have returned to normal, resistive loading and stretching of the elbow can be performed.

Complete recovery occurs in 88% of all operated cases and return to pre-injury state takes 3-6 months.

Chapter 8) Complications of epicondylitis.

Epicondylitis is a common condition with problems that linger. It is of great importance that physicians and all medical professionals involved in diagnosing and treating diseases be acquainted with this condition. A miss diagnosis can be functionally grave to a patient and so can mistaking another medical condition for tennis or golfer's elbow. The longer the condition is left untreated, the more likely it is to lead to chronicity, which actually never resolves. This chronicity comes with long-lasting pain, which restricts movement in day-to-day life activities such as opening doors, gripping handles and carrying things. This will eventually lead to loss of function and loss of dependence besides, which an even severe injury may occur.

Other complications are associated with the different kinds of epicondylitis treatment. Surgery for one may result in swelling, numbness, stiffness, and scar formation. Early physiotherapy of fingers and elevating the limb can reduce its severity. In most patients swelling greatly decreases by the end of the first week, though local incision swelling may persist resulting in a scar or even keloid. Infection, though rare, estimated at less than 1% of all operated cases of epicondylitis may occur. These infections can be treated by oral or intravenous antibiotics, depending on severity. A neuroma is defined as a painful bundle of nerve tissue, also found in less than a percent of all cases treated with surgery. Failure of surgery is yet another complication which necessitates reoperation, exposing the patient to double doses of anaesthesia and surgical associated risks. Reflex sympathetic dystrophy (RSD), pain and muscle wasting occurring on the hands whether the surgery was minor or major may develop. 2% is estimated to be its occurrence. Radioulnar joint dysfunction or instability in tennis elbow causes degeneration with consequent arthritis development, pain even in the absence of any soft tissue injury, and is the main cause of chronicity and recurrence. Nerve damage is possible, especially to the small nerves that supply the skin. This results in loss of sensation on specific zones of the elbow. Injury to the ligaments, in particular the lateral collateral ligament, will require more surgery. Other complications involve the incorrect use of elbow braces, resulting in pressure sores, joint stiffness or cut-off blood supply.

Chapter 8) Complications of epicondylitis

Chapter 9) Where To Get Help.

Remember, any information contained in this book is not to replace advice from a doctor, hence your physician is the first person to turn to when you have any medical complaints including tennis elbow or golfer's elbow-associated complaints especially if they are acute. This is important as your physician will do a general examination and imaging or laboratory investigations to rule out any immediate danger, which can result in a very fatal outcome. If it is truly tennis or golfer's elbow, depending on your doctor's experience, he or she may initiate treatment and/or refer you to the right specialist.

Another way to do this is to make an appointment directly with a specialist. Specialists like othorpaedic surgeons, sports medicine doctors, physiotherapists and rheumatologists do understand and have experience with tennis and golfer's elbow. The Internet is one way to locate the closest unit in your area, offering the above named specialties; otherwise you can also call the directory for assistance. Google Maps is one tool to find directions to a specific hospital or centre if known, and also, if not known, on Google Maps one can enter a location, and then search for sports medicine or physiotherapy in that particular area. A centre within your reach will appear with even directions on how to get there. Making an appointment is always good before going there because walk-in services at times result in unnecessary delays especially in big busy centres.

While in the process of locating a prospective treatment executer, it doesn't necessarily mean that you cannot initiate treatment. This is why reader's guides like this particular book are written- for the sole purpose of educating the reader. After reading through earlier chapters, your knowledge at present is adequate for you to self-assist. You can start by stopping the symptom-stimulating activity, though not completely stopping function of the joint, as some form of activity is still required. Take over-the-counter pain medicines such as Tylenol and initiate the RICE method. Elevating the affected limb can help reduce swelling and pain. Elbow orthotics like braces, splints, supports and straps are also introduced during the day or at night to help relieve tension on the affected tendon. These are available from sporting shops and online outlets like Amazon.com or Amazon.co.uk. eBay is another source and preference of a supplier should be based on other customers' reviews. Other source websites include bodybraces.co.uk, medibrace.com, and isokineticsinc.com. Points to note on how to choose the correct brace for your elbow are explained under physiotherapy and rehabilitation topics.

Knowledge is power – it's true and the more knowledge you accumulate on a problem, the sooner you can find a solution. Read more books on tennis or golfer's elbow, for instance Jim Johnson's *Treat your own tennis elbow* book available on Amazon. Books of technique are also useful such as learning how to maintain correct posture in *Defying the pains of gravity: Using proper posture technique* by Jeff LaBianco, a doctor of physical therapy and certified strength and conditioning specialist, also available on Amazon. *Biomechanical principles of tennis technique: Using science to improve your strokes* by Duane V. Khudson, and *Athletic and sports issues in musculoskeletal rehabilitation* by David J. Magee, Robert C. Manske, James E. Zachazewski and William S. Quillen are also excellent reads especially for those involved in more than one sporting activity, as these books explain what to do and not to do when exercising in specific sports such as golf, tennis, swimming, cycling, etc.

Further understanding can be acquired by joining tennis elbow or golfer's elbow discussion groups. Here, people share their

73

experiences, success stories and failed medical trials. Discussion groups, for instance, 'Tennis warehouse," have a wide range of discussion topics going on, from the best equipment choices such as strings, rackets and even techniques giving sources of where one can get them from. Google group discussions and tennis elbow CrossFit discussion boards are amongst the listed.

Websites such as WebMD, webtennis.net, tenniselbowdoctor.com, orthoinfo.aaos.org, royalberkshire.nhs.uk, nismat.org, livestrong.com, health1949.com, sure-health.co.uk, to mention just a few, are great sources for further short and precise education on tennis and golfer's elbow. Exercise routines are best learned via video and can be found on YouTube.

The thinking behind it is that a patient who understands their medical condition deeply is a disease halfway cured.

Chapter 10) Physiotherapy

a) What is physio?

When someone is affected by injury, illness or disability, physiotherapy helps to restore function. Physiotherapy is the same as rehabilitation through three disciplines - physical rehabilitation (rehab), physical therapy (PT) and occupational therapy (OT) are used to manage injury, illness or disability for maintenance and function restoration. Physiotherapy is a branch of medicine, a science in its own right, which approaches health and well-being of a patient by taking into account the person as a whole, including his/her general lifestyle. It uses natural methods such as exercise, motivation, advocacy, education and evidence-based routines to treat a variety of conditions that affect physical ability in both adults and children. Physiotherapists are professionals who are trained to perform physiotherapy and during their training they learn the human body in topics like anatomy, physiology, neurology and developmental milestones. This knowledge is then used to improve a range of medical conditions associated with different body systems, such as neuromuscular, musculoskeletal, respiratory, and cardiovascular conditions. Physiotherapists can be found in hospital wards, clinics, schools, sports centres and specialist units as well as in the community where they can visit a patient in the comfort of their home for treatment.

b) What do I consider when looking for a physiotherapist?

By law, physiotherapists are required to be registered and certified by the physiotherapy board, in the United Kingdom, the Health and Care Professions Council (HCPC), while in the U.S., the Federation of State Boards of Physical Therapy (FSBPT). It is also required that a physiotherapist renew their license on a regular basis, with a majority of states requiring continuing education for a renewal. It is important therefore, when choosing a personal therapist for your tennis/golfer's elbow to confirm credibility and this can be done by searching the physiotherapist's name on hcpc-uk.org. Here in the U.K. chartered physiotherapists are recommended, that is they have MCSP after their name.

A therapist with many years of work has more experience and one should remember to ask their therapist's experience before making an appointment, and those who completed a residency or fellowship in orthopaedic physical therapy have advanced knowledge and skill in golfer's/tennis elbow. Other miscellaneous tips include consideration of therapist recommendations by friends, family and/or health care providers.

c) How can I find a physiotherapist?

Two main types of physiotherapist exist at your disposal and these are private practitioners and those available via the NHS system. Finding either one closest to your location is an added advantage for many reasons. To locate a physiotherapist, visit www.csp.org.uk, where you select the Health tab and choose Physio2u. Using a full postcode, you can find contact information for a chartered therapist near your home. Another option that you could use to search for a therapist is via physiofirst.org.uk. The American Physical Therapy Association (APTA) on www.apta.org has devised a "Find a PT" online tool where using a postcode or city you can locate a physical therapist.

Before taking any physio sessions, if you have medical insurance, check whether you are eligible, but most private medical insurance schemes often include physiotherapy.

Chapter 10) Physiotherapy

Chapter 11) Tennis/Golfer's Elbow Exercises

a) Why exercise?

You do not have to go to expensive physical therapists or waste money on private gym training; you do not require expensive equipment either. Epicondylitis can be cured at home if you know and understand some exercise programs for your condition. Exercises are an important phase of treatment for epicondylitis and to date, several routines have been formulated worldwide. They are designed to strengthen muscles in the forearm and to increase stretch flexibility at the elbow joint. Each routine is usually repeated five times a day on a daily or alternate day basis. If done correctly, in most cases, relief of pain is first noticed after four to six weeks. Otherwise, a bad technique on a bad elbow is a recipe for disaster.

Before discussing any specific exercise routines, it is relevant to point out that a correct elbow environment is necessary for optimal healing and benefit from exercise. Nutrients, elements and water should be in the right quantities and of particular reference is omega-3 supplementing, which is known to reduce inflammation and prevent tendon scarring. If it is, however, not possible to get omega-3 supplements, one can include them in their diet from fish, chia seeds, walnuts, wild rice, canola oil, flax seeds and omega-3-enriched dairy foods. Adequate blood supply at the elbow can be generated by warm presses and massage. This causes blood vessels to dilate, increasing the flow of blood to elbow tissues. Massage also aids in balancing muscles and releasing any soft tissue restrictions. Professional masseuses are somewhat expensive for daily therapy. One can substitute by using daily self-myofascial release (SMR) gadgets such as foam rollers and trigger point therapy (TPT) on biceps, triceps, the upper back and upper chest. The more the whole body can move in sync, the better the elbow will feel. This is also the same concept used for exercise choice. Exercises targeting the whole body, for instance, pull-ups and push-ups, which generally strengthen the upper body are preferred to those tackling single muscle groups or joints such as bicep curls and shoulder flies.

Tendon healing is a very slow process and controversies on when to introduce exercise as a treatment for epicondylitis is a daily specialist dilemma. Others talk of rest and wait it out, after which they introduce exercise routines. This technique to me is a waste of time because stalling for a few weeks does relieve pain, but as soon as exercise commences, so does the pain. It's almost like you are still in the position where you were at the beginning. Then, other specialists prefer starting exercise at once, a no pain, no gain approach. Vigorous activity can worsen acute epicondylitis, leading to lingering of the disease. From my experience, I prefer neither waiting it out nor early vigorous routine initiation. I follow the three-phase treatment plan described under chapter six where I prescribe non-steroidal anti-inflammatory drugs, use the RICE method and at the same time with an elbow support do a gentle stretch to improve the quality of tissues in the elbow. This particular stretch I almost always use for all my patients and is called the elbow and wrist flexors stretch. With an extended elbow of the affected limb, palm facing forward, gently use the healthy hand to pull fingers of the ill side backward into a greatly extended wrist, holding the position for two minutes, and then releasing and repeating the same process with fingers down into greater flexion. With this exercise, one can feel a pulling on both flexors and extensors of the forearm, rejuvenating and maintaining typical muscle movement. This is to be done about five times a day with three times rotation in a single routine.

Walking, jogging, water aerobics and cycling improve the circulatory system, heart and lungs, thus increasing endurance and further maximizing blood supply to the elbow. This fitness program I call the "pain shield", since patients concentrate more on the fitness activity and temporarily forget about the elbow pain. There is a group of certain individuals who experience muscle spasms. To them, local elbow ultrasound therapy is added at a dose of ten minutes per session done five times over two weeks.

As the muscles build strength, routine exercises are then begun, gradually increasing intensity or toughness at an interval of three weeks. This means that when a routine is started, it is maintained for three weeks, after which a different, slightly more tough routine is started, also being maintained for another three weeks before a change. This climbing a ladder approach allows for the elbow to adjust adequately at every level before gradually being exposed to an even more intense force. This is done for about three to six months, a period during which it's expected for any elbow pain or discomfort to have disappeared.

Approaches differ, however; other specialists introduce a set of five, maybe seven different exercises to be done one after another in a single routine repeated over three times daily. This also seems to be effective as tennis or golfer's elbow physiotherapy treatment plans.

b) The importance of stretching

Stretching exercises encourage muscle and tendon lengthening to normalize the muscle length tension ratio. This is contrary to what many people imagine muscle contraction to be, i.e. contraction and shortening witnessed in vigorous exercises or for a simple example as seen in making a bicep hump. These two types of contractions produce different effects on the body depending on the targeted outcome. For a healthy athlete who requires bulk, stamina and physique, vigorous exercises are his bit, but for an epicondylitis sufferer who is under rehabilitation, muscle lengthening with contraction is the way to go. Lengthening muscles by stretching promotes flexibility and complete range of motion about a joint, though only if the stretching is done in the correct way.

c) How to stretch properly

Those who have watched Olympics live or on the television might have noticed that sportsmen stretch in their tracksuits before competing. Their stretches range from a simple on-the-spot up and down jumping to limb straightening manipulations. This is of utmost importance, because muscles should only be stretched when they are warm; cold muscles have a greater chance of tearing. Stretching differs depending on the endpoint expected effect, as in, is it a stretch before exercise, at the end of an exercise routine, to recover from an exercise and/or to rehabilitate from injury. Before engaging in any exercise routine, warm up your muscles by jumping in place for approximately 5 minutes and/or a light 5-minute jog. After warm–up, one then starts slow static stretches ideally for 20-30 seconds. For epicondylitis, whether medial or lateral, a simple elbow and wrist flexors stretch will suffice. Modify the intensity by gradually increasing speed and power to the correct force required for your intended final exercise. Only after this preparation, should exercise commence. After the exercise, one should also stretch, and this should cover most of your stretching time around 5-10 minutes, concentrating on the muscles that you have just exercised. This is done to help return your muscles to their resting state, at the same time preparing them for your next exercise session.

d) Eccentric exercises

Eccentric elbow exercises are the cornerstone of epicondylitis treatment and they can be performed in many styles using all kinds of equipment. This movement comprises of muscle fiber lengthening and contraction as in extending the elbow while holding a weight. To get better results from performing eccentric exercises for your tennis or golfer's elbow, there is some knowledge you are required to grasp. First and foremost are the three principles governing the eccentric loading regimes:

1) Length of a tendon - if a tendon is pre-stretched by warm-up before actual eccentric exercise, its resting length increases, thus less strain will be necessary to produce movement.

2) Load - progressively increasing load weight increases the inherent tendon strength.

3) Speed - greater force will develop by increasing the speed of eccentric contractions.

Eccentric training is a powerful tool for tennis and golfer's elbow treatment; it increases flexibility, tendon strength and bulk, producing greater hypertrophy with faster routines all for a little energy. One is stronger when they perform eccentric exercises than with any other kind. Muscles have three types of contractions: eccentric, concentric and isometric. During eccentric phase of any lift, you are about 1.75 times stronger than in concentric phase. On eccentric muscle contractions, remember to control the downward force if you are to fully benefit from the exercise, never allow gravity to do the job for you. Any exercise is therefore lowered in a slow pace usually over four to six seconds. Any fast lowering or pull can damage tendons and muscles by overstretch. However, when power is the desired effect of these exercises, they have to be done at a fast speed.

The right intensity load is required for proper tendon/muscle stimulation. Too heavy a load can lead to overstrain and fiber damage

e) Normal movement at the elbow joint

Movement at the elbow or wrist havw specific terms used by physiotherapists and specialists which are of importance to your understanding any context in which they are to be used throughout this book. If one is to follow instructions of exercise routines, a correct knowledge of these movements is required. These are supination, pronation, abduction, adduction, flexion and extension. As you might notice, they exist in pairs because most are opposites. Supination of the forearm occurs when the forearm is rotated in such a way that the palm faces up. Pronation is the opposite of that, involving rotating the forearm to face the palm down. Supination and pronation are made possible by the proximal and distal radius-to-ulna articulations in the forearm where the radius is the only mobile bone rotating on the ulna. Abduction is a movement that brings a body part closer to the middle, for instance, when you tuck the upper limb close to the body. Adduction, therefore, means movement away from the middle, an example being raising the arm on the side to shoulder level. Flexion is another movement; it involves bending a joint to decrease the angle of its articulations. Elbow flexion is appreciated when you touch the shoulder, while wrist flexion by an attempt to touch the forearm with fingers. Extension, being the opposite of flexion, means increasing the angle at a joint, straightening the elbow and a high five for the wrist. It is very important to grasp these movements for a better understanding of specific tests and stretch exercises to be encountered throughout the book.

f) Stretch exercises for tennis/golfers elbow

1) Tennis ball squeeze exercise

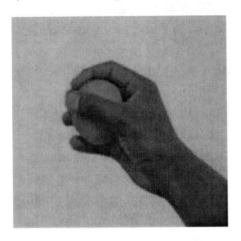

1) With the affected limb hold a tennis ball.

2) Tightly squeeze the ball 20-25 times.

3) Repeat step 2 to make 3 sets, resting 30 seconds in between each set.

Tip:

If your elbow is too tender, use a sponge or something softer and then gradually increase the stiffness.

2) Clockwise/Counterclockwise twist

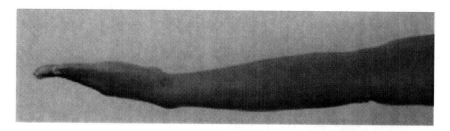

1) Stand in an upright position with the arm straight in front of you.

2) Rotate the whole arm in a clockwise direction to the maximum degree that you can and hold the position for 20 seconds.

3) Then, rotate it in a counterclockwise direction again to the maximum degree possible, holding for 20 seconds.

4) Repeat the rotations 20-25 times

5) Do 3 sets of 20-25 rotations a set, with 1 minute rest between each set. To be done daily, from several weeks to months.

3) Rubber band stretches

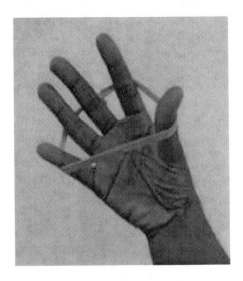

1) Place a rubber band over the fingers and thumb.

2) Open your hand as wide as possible stretching the rubber band in the process.

3) Repeat this process in 3 sets of 20 repetitions, 4-5 times a day.

Tip:

A stretch is felt on the elbow. Finding a suitable rubber band for your routine is challenging. They can be acquired from Amazon.com. If your desired size is not available, substitute with elastic hair bands and/or ask your physiotherapist for help on finding a suitable elastic band for your exercise.

4) 180° elbow stretch

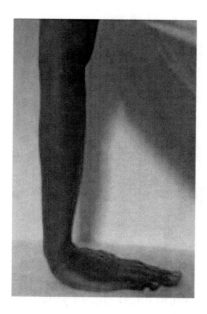

1) Rest your palm on the table top in a reverse 180° position, such that your fingers are facing you.

2) Gradually lean your body backwards to a tolerable stretch and hold the position for about 30 seconds. You will feel a deep stretch on the elbow anterior and forearm muscles. Do not overstretch.

3) Release by leaning forward and repeat the process for about 10 times, 5 times a day from several weeks to months.

5) Massage

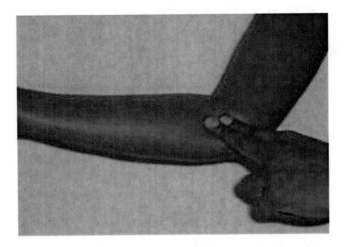

1) Locate the tender spot on your elbow.

2) Apply firm pressure using the index and tall finger of your normal hand.

3) Rub for 5 minutes in circular motion over the tender spot.

Repeat whenever required.

6) Golfers elbow stretch

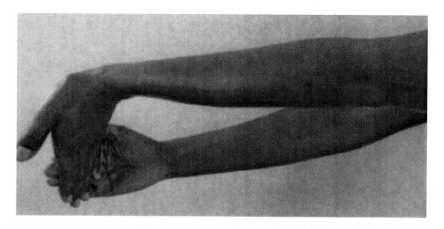

1) Stand upright, with your elbow stretched like a policeman stopping a car.

2) Rotate the fingers to point downwards.

3) Pull the fingers towards yourself into a mild to moderate stretch using the normal hand, and hold that position for 30 seconds.

4) Release the hold and repeat 4 times.

Can be done 3-5 times daily

7) Elbow flexion extension stretch

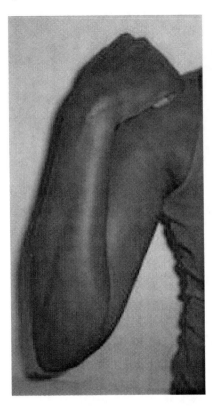

1) Bend and stretch the affected limb out as far as you can.

2) Stretching moderately.

3) Repeat 10-20 times provided the exercise is pain free.

8) Forearm rotation exercise

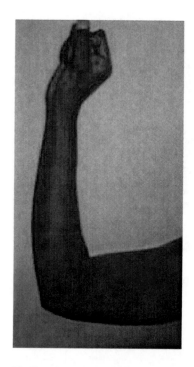

1) Get in a standing position, with a 90° flexed elbow.

2) Rotate the forearm clockwise and counterclockwise (supinate and pronate) as far as you can without pain.

3) Repeat this process 10-20 times.

9) Advanced elbow extension stretch

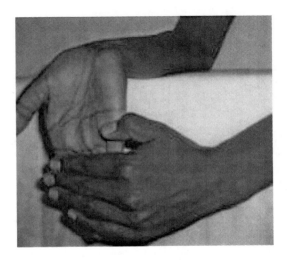

1) Use the affected side, supinated straight over the table, with the wrist hanging over for step 2.

2) Pull the forearm down the edge of the table, stretching as far as you can.

3) Hold the position for 30 seconds and repeat the process 10-20 times.

10) Advance elbow flexion

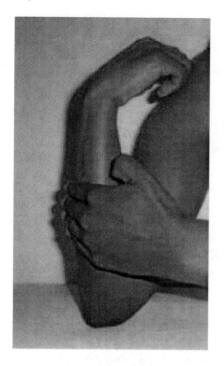

1) Using the affected limb on a flat surface, such as a table top, flex your elbow as far as you can.

2) Using the normal hand, pull on the flexed elbow towards you to a moderate stretch.

3) Hold the position for 30 seconds and repeat the process 10 times.

11) Advanced bicep stretch

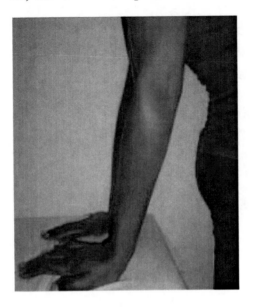

1) Stand in front of a table, with your back towards it.

2) Extend your forearms behind you, such that you touch the table behind.

3) Place your hands with an extended wrist position, maintaining the extension of the elbow.

4) Gently lower your body, allowing your forearms to move further behind you, until you feel a mild to a moderate stretch.

5) Hold for 30 seconds and release by pulling your body up.

6) Repeat the process 4 times.

12) Advanced triceps stretch

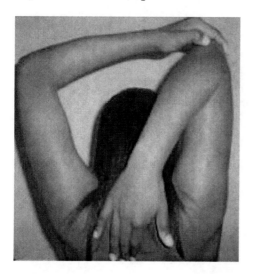

1) Using affected limb, touch the opposite shoulder from behind your head.

2) Moving your hand forward, use the normal hand to pull on the elbow of the affected side to a stretch.

3) Stretch mildly-moderately, as far as you can.

4) Hold for 30 seconds and release.

5) Repeat the procedure 4 times.

13) Wrist flexion extension exercise

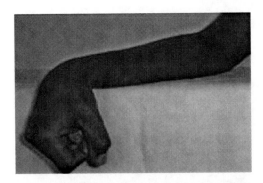

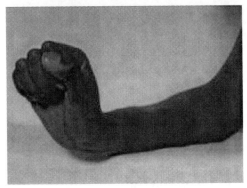

1) Place the affected limb, with forearm and fist facing down, on a table or bench.

2) Dangle your wrist over the table edge.

3) Bend your wrist forwards and backwards, as far as you can, to a mild-moderate stretch.

4) Repeat 10 times.

14) Wrist side bends

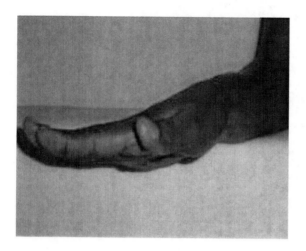

1) Using the affected limb, place your forearm to lie over a table top or bench.

2) Hold your fingers together in a straight position over the edge.

3) Move your wrist to one side, holding the position with a stretch for 30 seconds.

4) Move your wrist to the other side and stretch for another 30 seconds.

5) Repeat the cycle 10 times.

15) Wall tennis elbow stretch

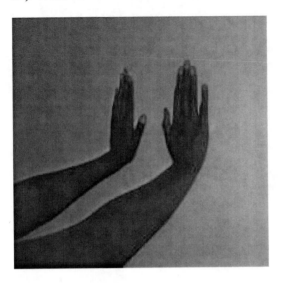

1) Stretch both arms out in front of you. Place your palms flat on a wall, fingers facing up.

2) Lift the base of your palms, such that only the fingers are up against the wall

3) Move your feet a few steps back without shifting the hand position.

4) With your body in a slanted position, press down gently moving your body up and down like push ups.

5) Repeat push ups 10 times, only if pain free.

16) Fancy forearm and elbow stretch

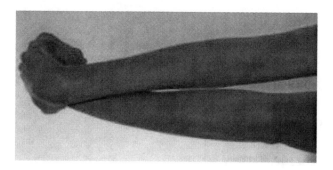

For the following exercise, if you have an affected right arm, follow the procedure as below. If left is affected, switch the arm positions.

1) Stand in a relaxed position and extend both arms before you.

2) Put your right arm over the left and interweave your fingers together.

3) With your left hand pull the right hand upwards, keeping the arms locked at the elbow.

4) Hold this stretch for 30-40 seconds, then release. Repeat 3-4 times daily.

Tip:

Readily available home equipment can be used, such as a broomstick, a full soda can in place of dumbbells, a baked potato as heat therapy, etc. These exercises additionally intensify an exercise routine.

17) Broomstick stretch

1) Using the affected hand, grip the middle of a broomstick in a vertical position, hand stretched out before you.

2) Move the broom forward into a horizontal position.

3) Bring it back up to the starting position.

4) Repeat the process 10 times.

Tip:

To increase the intensity of this exercise, tighten your grip at the lower end of the broomstick, so more weight is applied on the stretch by the broomstick.

18) Dumbbell elbow stretch

1) Using the affected hand, grip the lower end of the dumbbell.

2) Position the dumbbell into a vertical position, stretched out before you.

3) Lower the dumbbell into a horizontal position and hold for 30 seconds.

4) Bring the dumbbell back up to a vertical position.

5) Rest for 5 seconds and repeat the procedure again. To be done 10 times.

Tip:

Increasing the intensity of any stretch can be done by using devices designed for particular exercise routines. These devices include, Thera Band Flexbar, resistance bands, dumbbells, and physio elastic rubber bands to mention a few.

19) Ribbed pliable bars

Ribbed pliable bars e.g. Thera Band Flex bar, are twelve-inch long bars made from natural rubber. They are durable devices with a ridged surface for a non-slippery grip during use. Thera Band Flex bar is made in four consecutive resistant levels to match user capability. The yellow colored bar requires six pounds of force to bend into a u-shape, red ten pounds, green fifteen and, the most challenging is blue at twenty-five pounds. They are available on amazon.co.uk at a price range between fourteen and eighteen pounds.

How to use Thera Band Flex bar:

a) Using the affected limb, hand, wrist and elbow fully extended, hold the distal end of the bar, keeping it in a vertical position.

b) With the healthy side, firmly hold the proximal end of the bar to form a tight grip.

c) Twist the bar with the normal hand to a horizontal position with the wrist flexed.

d) Straighten the bar in an untwisting movement using the affected side, maintaining the grip.

e) Repeat the twisting and untwisting movement of the bar over four seconds each time, making three sets of fifteen daily, with thirty seconds rest between each set.

This is an eccentric exercise, meaning that muscle fibers contract and lengthen simultaneously. Unlike bicep curls, which are concentric, the muscle fibers contract and shorten. Since 1986, eccentric exercises have been used for tennis elbow treatment. It is thought that effective lengthening of the muscle tendon complex causes tendon remodeling with hypertrophy, an ultimate increase in tensile strength. Eccentric exercises are also known to provide central adaptation to opposing muscle groups, agonist and antagonist, therefore further improving function during rehabilitation.

Studies, which were conducted using flex bar eccentric exercises, have shown that symptom resolutions have occurred at an average of seven weeks, in ten separate clinics. This is actually impressive, for tennis elbow treatment can be a pain, lasting from over six months to even two years.

Flex bar exercises are also used for golfer's elbow treatment, but the steps on how to use the bar are somewhat in a reverse position.

a) The affected hand holds the proximal end of the bar facing downwards.

b) Then, the normal hand holds the distal end of the bar with a firm grip.

c) Maintaining the grip, lower the bar to a horizontal position, with elbows straight.

d) Release the twist in the bar with the affected side, over four seconds.

e) Repeat the process of twisting and untwisting to make three sets of fifteen daily, with thirty seconds rest between each. This is to be done for six weeks. About seventy five to eighty five percent of sufferers who have used this method have seen remarkable results.

For a visual on flex bar use, on YouTube look up "Tennis elbow: Step by Step Instructions for Treating Elbow Pain Using a Flexbar" by Austin Spine and Sport.

20) Dumbbell strengthening eccentric exercise

Using small size dumbbells of about three or five pounds, brace your forearm over a table top or any platform which allows forearm bracing.

a) Using the affected limb, with an extended arm, flex your wrist over the table top. Flex the wrist like you are attempting to touch the forearm with a dumbbell.

b) Keep your forearm completely still and perform about twenty wraps.

c) Turn your forearm backwards and perform the same exercise, only this time, extending the wrist again, making twenty wraps.

d) Add a side to side movement for another twenty wraps.

Repeat this exercise in three sets of twenty each daily, for six weeks. Visit YouTube and search for "Strengthening exercises: How to Strengthen Tennis Elbow" by livestrong.

Argos, Walmart, Dick's Sporting Goods, and Sports Authority are all sources where you can buy dumbbells.

21) Wrist extensor glides by Mulligan

The fact that tennis or golfer's elbow is predictable and consistent on pain provocation and symptoms, means that specialists can develop a lot of different manipulations for the forearm flexor and extensor tendons as treatment regiments. One of these regiments is the wrist extensor glide by Mulligan. It is a simple and affordable exercise, which only requires tape, indicated for tennis elbow with resistance upon extending the wrist.

1) The examiner locates the painful point on the extensor muscle group.

2) Using both thumbs, glide the extensor muscle group laterally.

3) The patient is asked to extend the wrist, while the examiner laterally glides the muscle group. The moment it becomes pain free, an assistant helps by applying a 5 centimeter wide strip of tape over the extensor muscles, 2-3 centimeters below the elbow in a lateral direction, ensuring the tape does not completely wrap the forearm.

4) The examiner repeats the lateral glide with both thumbs as before and the assistant reinforces the tape by firmly attaching another strip over it.

For a visual, see YouTube "Mulligan Taping Techniques: Tennis Elbow" by itherapies.

22) Resistance band therapy

A resistance band is a thick elastic rope, which has handles on either end.

1) Fix the resistance band under your foot (preferably mid foot, to prevent the rope from sliding out during the exercise).

2) With a straight elbow of the affected side, hold the rope in such a way that the hand in a fist lies in an extended position above, aligned to the knee.

3) Place the normal hand over the fist of the affected side.

4) Let the wrist of the affected side slowly drop towards the floor over 4 seconds.

5) Use the normal hand to pull the affected side back to the starting point.

6) Release the normal hand and let the affected side wrist to drop again, slowly towards the floor. This marks a single cycle of this particular exercise. Repeat the process 15 times, then rest for a minute after which you repeat 2 sets of 15. To be done daily about 3-5 times, from several weeks to months.

Modifications to the exercise are that you can harden the process by using a shorter or stiffer band. Work faster to improve bulk once you are used to the session and if there is no pain.

Heavy grips hand grippers

Heavy grips are high quality aluminum handled hand-clippers which are made starting with 50 pound increments, to 100 pounds of tension, to the maximum of 350 pounds. This trains the forearm by increasing resistance in a movement, similar to gripping pliers. For beginners, HG100 is recommended and then you work your way up. Training both upper limbs - affected or not, is recommended to maintain muscular balance, always starting with the normal one. This exercise is introduced for when the pain hasn't been felt for several months and muscular strength is almost returned to its old self. Heavy grippers can be bought online at heavygrips.com, leehayward.com, or eBay.com.

23) Swiss ball exercises

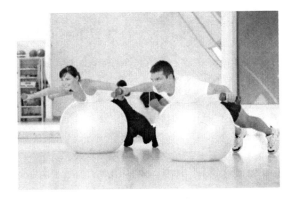

Swiss balls are handy exercise equipment that can be used singularly or in a combination with dumbbells for an intense exercise routine. Many websites have Swiss balls available including, www.ball-express.com, www.self.com, www.healthyliving.azcentral.com, www.workoutbox.com, and these are just a few. www.Tracker.dailyburn.com offers some exercise programs using a Swiss ball. Try out this stretch.

1) Lie on a Swiss ball, with your chest and arms stretched out as if you are flying.

2) Stretch your arms backwards and hold for 30 seconds.

3) Release and repeat the process 10 times.

Tip:

If your elbow is not too tender, you can do this exercise while holding small dumbbells. This exercise can be done in reverse too, with your back on the Swiss ball.

Chapter 12) Elbow Braces

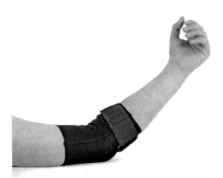

a) What is a brace?

Since growing up I remember braces used to be worn specifically for protection to prevent future injuries, somehow they have evolved in the past decades. Tennis/golfer's elbow bands are over-the-counter devices sold under different names such as counterforce brace, elbow strap, elbow support, forearm support band, elbow clasp, elbow sleeve and magnetic elbow brace. They are described as flexible wraps that fit well around the forearm below the elbow joint providing pressure to underlying tissues. Tennis elbow straps are reported by many patients to be helpful. They are designed to be worn 2-3 centimeters from the elbow. This position is intended to lift stress off the tendon on its point of attachment at the epicondyle. Straps are not used as a primary treatment plan, but as a supplement when one is stretching and/or exercising.

b) How do they work?

The easiest way to understand how straps function is to imagine strumming on a guitar. When one strums a tune on a guitar the strings vibrate along their entire length. If a hand is placed in the middle to compress the strings on the fret bar, tension is applied in such a way that the lengths of the strings shorten in either direction from the point where the hand is placed. One part of the strings closest to the guitar body moves, producing a high pitch tone while the one farthest does not. Imagining this, if applied to strap function, the area under the strap acts as a new muscle pivot dividing extensor or flexor muscles into two parts. From the wrist to the band muscles can contract and function, whilst from the band to the elbow there is no movement. This allows the muscle portion from the band to the elbow to rest and in this particular fashion pain is usually relieved.

Research on the use of straps has, however, been largely inconclusive, with studies showing that a tennis elbow band can reduce force on muscle attachment at the elbow by 13-15% throughout a range of different activities. So, wearing a band actually has an impact on stress distribution in the forearm. Long-term strap use outcomes are not known, but bracing for over 6 weeks has been shown to improve performance.

Elbow braces are relatively inexpensive and can be purchased in pharmacies, sporting goods stores and online outlets. They cost from as little as $5 to more depending on the brand. Even though no guarantees exist by evidence, just the worthwhile thought of a possibility is enough for a trial. You never know, you might actually remain active through your epicondylitis.

c) Effective elbow straps

From different patients' perspectives the most effective forearm bands are the ones with padding underneath, be it silicon padding or cotton. It is reported that they reduce pressure on the affected tendon without scraping uncomfortably on the skin and tissues below to cause a pressure sore. Another group of sufferers reported that the elbow straps with an air bubble work very well because it puts pressure on the tendon more than the entire arm and that this bubble greatly affects its performance. It is required, however, that one finds the sore tendon or assign a physical therapist to look at it if it is to be worn in the correct optimal position. PneuGel tennis elbow support from DeRoyal is an example and with this particular one a patient has the ability to pump the air bubble themselves to vary levels of air tension, and also the air bubble can be placed in a freezer. Tommie Copper elbow compression sleeves are another excellent choice found at about $30 on tommiecopper.com. They are comfortable fabric elbow supports made from 57% copper-nylon, 24% nylon, and 14% spandex. They have several advantages, such as anti-odor technology, wick-able fabric which keeps skin dry, they are machine-washable and available in a wide array of colours and come in all sizes. Websites where more braces can be found are flexcart.com, adidas.com, mcdavidusa.com, tennis-warehouse.com and uk.tennis-elbowbrace.com.

Counterforce tennis/golfer's elbow straps are effective for use during an activity such as playing tennis through your epicondylitis as they produce more grip strength with less pain.

Magnetic elbow wraps are superior in terms of pain relief. One study had sufferers placed into two groups. One group was given magnetic elbow wraps and the other general regular elbow wear. The group that had magnetic wraps, reported more pain relief by over three-quarters. Magnets are gauss units, i.e. their strength is measured in gauss. Fridge magnets are less than 50 gauss and about 1,000 gauss are required for one to reach a therapeutic gauss level. The more the gauss, the deeper the magnetic strength reaches and the more the pain relief. Pain relief is, however, not instantaneous, but positive effects have been reported in as little as 2 weeks. There are no side effects to their use, but for people with metallic implants, a doctor consultation may be required.

Another technique is to use a strap on a totally different location to the one under therapy. For example, for epicondylitis shoulder and wrist braces are also widely used. Wrist braces are worn at the wrist to keep the wrist bent backwards to take stress off muscles as they insert at the wrist. These can be additions in cases where pain is severe and other measures have failed. Wrist braces are, however, used mostly during the night, but can be used during the day as well.

Due to research by patients and professionals, many have discovered that different types of straps are effective at varying times. For instance, when working out, a counterforce strap is preferred in comparison to a padded forearm band, which is the option of choice at rest. Size has not been shown to be of importance, but most straps used in multiple studies are between 5-8 centimeters in width. It is therefore recommended to consider using a strap of that width so as to avoid conflicting with the literatures.

Now that you probably have an elbow support or brace, are you using it correctly? The technique upon which elbow straps are used can influence it to either function as required or to cause further damage. Too tight a strap and application of pressure on the wrong points, are the two things that should be avoided during application of a strap. This can cut off blood supply to the forearm and elbow muscles and tendons as well as inadequately compress on the tendon as it should. Here is how to properly use these devices:

d) How to wear a tennis elbow support

1) Palpate on the lateral epicondyle to locate the most tender spot

2) Slide the tennis elbow support over the affected elbow

3) Position the support in such a way that the cushioned part lies on top of the most tender spot, located in step 1

4) Wrap the adjustable straps around the forearm to keep it in place, though not tight for a comfortable, firm fit.

e) How to wear an elbow arm band

1) Place your affected elbow on a soft, cushioned surface such as a pillow

2) Palpate on the lateral epicondyle to locate the most tender area

3) Using your index finger and thumb span, estimate about 10 centimeters below the tender spot located in step 2

4) Place the brace component of the arm band directly over the tender spot, hanging the Velcro strap down your arm. Position the brace in such a way that the strap rests on the outside of the forearm

5) Hold the brace in place as you fasten the Velcro strap on top of the brace component

6) For lateral epicondylitis, the brace should be firmly wrapped around your arm, reinforcing the lateral muscles into a firm, comfortable fit. If you experience a tingling sensation or a sudden paleness in arms, your brace may be too tight and is occluding blood supply. Loosen the Velcro straps a bit.

f) Misconceptions

Lateral and medial epicondylitis are two different conditions, though they are both caused by RSIs. This should be noted, because a frequent misconception is that they can both be treated by the exact same brace and exercises. This is not the case. If one is suffering from lateral epicondylitis, the shock-absorbing strap pad is placed on the outside of the elbow or forearm, whereas in medial it stays on the inside.

g) How to wear a golfer's elbow brace

A typical golfer's elbow brace is a single elastic strap that wraps around the forearm. A metal D-ring and Velcro patch secure its fit.

1) Palpate the most tender spot on the medial elbow surface

2) Place the brace 2 finger breaths below the medial elbow crease, positioning the shock-absorbing pad above the tender spot found in step 1

3) Slip the elastic strap through the D-ring and fasten it back against itself.

Whether you have lateral or medial epicondylitis, finding the correct brace or support size is sometimes difficult. To prevent returns, especially if you buy them from online outlets like Amazon, measure in centimeters the widest part of your forearm, then consult with the brace packaging for the appropriate strap size.

h) Are we treating the real issue with a strap?

Although forearm braces are recommended everywhere you go, reasons exist as to why their use is a bad idea for treating epicondylitis no matter how good a brace might look, and its function is compared to none, if not worse. This is a myth, per se stating that braces are effective in treating and curing epicondylitis. The truth can only be realized upon closer inspection as to why they actually might hurt you instead. Firstly, wearing a splint indirectly causes less blood circulation. How? By restricting muscle, tendon and elbow joint movement, which compromises the more needed good blood and lymph flow.

Secondly, it directly compresses tissues and blood vessels, perturbing circulation. The tighter the brace, the more restrictive it is. Another downside is that when tissues are stuck together for long, adhesions and scars result, causing further restrictions and pain. As understood from previous topics, muscles, tendons and joints require constant movement to remain strong and/or to heal. A brace restricts movement, thus weakening these muscles and joints, worsening the condition. According to these controversies, elbow straps should only be used where there is an injury such as fracture or ligamentous sprain. However, the benefits reported by many are worth a try.

i) Tips

Do not use the braced limb to carry heavy stuff; always ask for assistance in such cases. Wear the brace/support for 4 weeks at a time. If by week 4 there is no relief, consult with your physician. Taking analgesics simultaneously often increases the extent of pain relief.

Summary

Epicondylitis is a common elbow complaint affecting mostly ages of 30-50 years. It affects both females and males at a ratio of 1:1, though studies have shown a little male dominance, which has no statistical significance. Medial epicondylitis (golfer's elbow) and lateral epicondylitis (tennis elbow) are two separate conditions, which result from the same mechanism of repeated tendon stress injuries in a background of tendinosis. These RSIs are often caused by sporting activities that involve repeated wrist flexion and extension, such as tennis, golf, baseball, and weightlifting. Sport is not the only causative factor, but day-to-day activities associated with professions like typing and meat cutting are uncommon. Epicondylitis common in society is of the chronic type with dominance of tennis elbow. General symptoms involve pain, tenderness, swelling and redness accentuated by resistance, stretch and grip. Specific symptoms are that in tennis elbow pain is felt on resisted wrist extension, wrist deviation towards the pinky, and palpated tenderness on the left epicondyle; in golfer's elbow resisted wrist flexion, on facing down the palm and palpation at the medial epicondyle. Tennis elbow has symptoms on the lateral elbow bony eminence whereas golfer's is on the medial, inner surface, the main difference not to be forgotten.

Diagnosis is usually done by specialists like physiotherapists, orthopaedic surgeons, sports medicine specialists and rheumatologists. General physical examination, with use of specific manipulative tests is the mainstay for diagnosis. Imaging such as X-rays, MRIs, CT scans and laboratory blood work like FBP, CRP and ESR plus specific functional tests of nerve conduction and muscle evaluation are necessary for differential diagnosis. Not only doctors can cure epicondylitis. Once the correct diagnosis has been made, one can do exercise programs and relieve pain by oneself at home with satisfactory results.

Treatment of epicondylitis involves three phases where different approaches are used interchangeably in combination and rarely alone. Cold and heat, NSAIDs, elbow bracing and natural therapies like acupuncture are used to reduce pain. Other intermediate therapies, such as ultrasound, magnetic therapy and shockwave treatment can be implemented and so can injections like autologous blood, Botox, glucose solution and cortisone. Eccentric exercises are used to maintain and/or regain forearm muscle function. Exercise works over several weeks and months of daily effort and, if not, of regular muscle challenging. If done correctly, sufferers usually achieve the required goal of pain elimination by 4-8 weeks with complete recovery at 3-6 months. Improper use of exercises and any other treatment programs might lead to chronicity, complications such as tendon tears and/or relapses. If, however, there is no relief in several weeks and/or if the pain seems to be worsening, consult your physician and consider surgery. Surgery usually takes a short time and is done as an outpatient procedure, but just as long as a patient is being given anaesthesia, surgical risks are always existent.

I hope this book has been adequately thorough in all required areas for one to better understand epicondylitis as a debilitating condition. With patience and endurance, your elbows can *smile* again.

Robert Rymore

Index

A

B

C

H

Osteopathy, **21**

P

Pannus. *See* vegetations
Pharmacological, **50**
Physiotherapy, **75**
plasma, **38**
Prolotherapy, **56**
Pronation, **83**
Pronator syndrome, **28**

R

Radial nerve, **27**
Radiculopathy, **21**
Radiographs, **32**
Radius, **8**
Reflex sympathetic dystrophy (RSD), **69**
repetitive stress injuries (RSIs), **9**
Resistance band, 105
Rheumatoid arthritis, **23**
RICE method, **79**

S

Self myofascial release (SMR), **78**
Stretching, **80**
Sublaxation, **12**
Supination, **83**
Swiss ball, **106**
Synovitis, **12**
Synovium, **12**

T

Tendinosis, **9**
Tendonitis. *See* tendinitis
Tennis elbow, 9, 10, 42, 43, 44, 46, 49, 58, 103, 108, 115
Thera Band Flex bar, **101**
Tinel sign, **28**
Trigger points, **21**